FIRST AID

The Boy Scouts of America is indebted to
the American Red Cross for its subject matter
expertise, review, and other assistance with
this edition of the *First Aid* merit badge pamphlet.

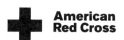

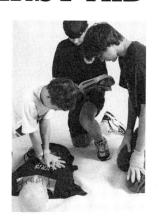

BOY SCOUTS OF AMERICA
IRVING, TEXAS

Requirements

1. Satisfy your counselor that you have current knowledge of all first-aid requirements for Tenderfoot, Second Class, and First Class ranks.

2. Do the following:

    a. Explain how you would obtain emergency medical assistance from your home, on a wilderness camping trip, and during an activity on open water.

    b. Explain the term *triage.*

    c. Explain the standard precautions as applied to bloodborne pathogens.

    d. Prepare a first-aid kit for your home. Display and discuss its contents with your counselor.

3. Do the following:

    a. Explain what action you should take for someone who shows signals of shock, for someone who shows signals of a heart attack, and for someone who shows signals of stroke.

    b. Identify the conditions that must exist before performing CPR on a person. Then demonstrate proper technique in performing CPR using a training device approved by your counselor.

    c. Explain the use of an automated external defibrillator (AED).

    d. Show the steps that need to be taken for someone suffering from a severe cut on the leg and on the wrist. Tell the dangers in the use of a tourniquet and the conditions under which its use is justified.

    e. Explain when a bee sting could be life threatening and what action should be taken for prevention and for first aid.

33301C
ISBN 978-0-8395-3301-6
©2007 Boy Scouts of America
2007 Printing

    f.   Explain the symptoms of heatstroke and what action should be taken for first aid and for prevention.

4. Do the following:

    a.   Describe the signals of a broken bone. Show first-aid procedures for handling fractures (broken bones), including open (compound) fractures of the forearm, wrist, upper leg, and lower leg using improvised materials.

    b.   Describe the symptoms and possible complications and demonstrate proper procedures for treating suspected injuries to the head, neck, and back. Explain what measures should be taken to reduce the possibility of further complicating these injuries.

5. Describe the symptoms, proper first-aid procedures, and possible prevention measures for the following conditions:

    a.   Hypothermia

    b.   Convulsions/seizures

    c.   Frostbite

    d.   Dehydration

    e.   Bruises, strains, sprains

    f.   Burns

    g.   Abdominal pain

    h.   Broken, chipped, or loosened tooth

    i.   Knocked out tooth

    j.   Muscle cramps

6. Do TWO of the following:

    a.   If a sick or an injured person must be moved, tell how you would determine the best method. Demonstrate this method.

    b.   With helpers under your supervision, improvise a stretcher and move a presumably unconscious person.

    c.   With your counselor's approval, arrange a visit with your patrol or troop to an emergency medical facility or through an American Red Cross chapter for a demonstration of how an AED is used.

7. Teach another Scout a first-aid skill selected by your counselor.

Contents

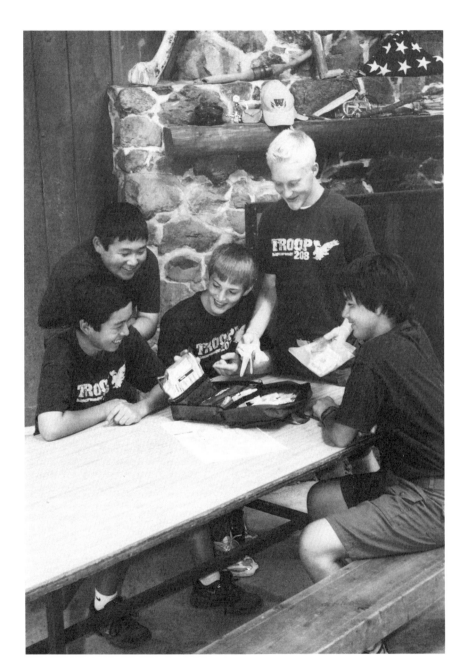

Introduction

First aid—caring for injured or ill persons until they can receive professional medical care—is an important skill for every Scout. With some knowledge of first aid, you can provide immediate care and help to someone who is hurt or who becomes ill. First aid can help prevent infection and serious loss of blood. It could even save a limb or a life.

The Goals of First Aid

- Protect a person who is injured or ill from further harm.
- Stop life-threatening medical emergencies. (Keep the airway open. Maintain breathing and circulation. Stop serious bleeding. Treat for shock.)
- Get the person under professional medical care.

First-aid requirements for the Tenderfoot, Second Class, and First Class ranks encourage you to practice treating certain injuries and ailments. Earning the First Aid merit badge will help you understand that emergency medical treatment is a set of clear action steps. By following the steps every time you come upon a first-aid emergency, you can quickly evaluate the situation, come up with a first-aid plan, and then see that plan through.

To learn how to treat for shock, see "How to Handle an Emergency."

First-Aid Rank Requirements

Tenderfoot

11. Identify local poisonous plants; tell how to treat for exposure to them.

12a. Demonstrate the Heimlich maneuver and tell when it is used.

12b. Show first aid for the following:

- Simple cuts and scratches
- Venomous snakebite
- Blisters on the hand and foot
- Nosebleed
- Minor burns or scalds (first-degree)
- Frostbite and sunburn
- Bites or stings of insects and ticks

Second Class

6a. Show what to do for "hurry" cases of stopped breathing, serious bleeding, and internal poisoning.

6b. Prepare a personal first-aid kit to take with you on a hike.

6c. Demonstrate first aid for the following:

- Object in the eye
- Bite of a suspected rabid animal
- Puncture wounds from a splinter, nail, and fishhook
- Serious burns (second-degree)
- Heat exhaustion
- Shock
- Heatstroke, dehydration, hypothermia, and hyperventilation

First Class

8b. Demonstrate bandages for a sprained ankle and for injuries on the head, the upper arm, and the collarbone.

8c. Show how to transport by yourself, and with one other person, a person

- From a smoke-filled room
- With a sprained ankle, for at least 25 yards

8d. Tell the five most common signs of a heart attack. Explain the steps (procedures) in cardiopulmonary resuscitation (CPR).

Reducing Risk

One way to stay healthy and safe both at home and when you are in the out-of-doors is to recognize that there is an element of risk in many activities. By being aware of risk and adjusting your behavior to manage it, you will also be in a stronger position to provide assistance should an emergency arise. Among the ways you can increase your role in risk management during Scouting adventures are the following:

- Stay in good physical condition so that you are ready for the demands of the activities you enjoy.

- Know where you are going and what to expect.

- Adjust clothing layers to match changing conditions.

- Drink plenty of water.

- Protect yourself from exposure to the sun, biting insects, and poisonous plants.

- Take care of your gear.

Scout troops and patrols can also manage risk as a group:

- Review and practice first-aid skills and techniques on a regular basis.

- Take responsibility for having a safe experience.

- Be sure everyone understands and follows group guidelines established to minimize risk.

- Ensure everyone has a say in recognizing and dealing with risks that might arise.

After you learn the first-aid skills and techniques required for the First Aid merit badge, you can teach another Scout what you have learned. Teaching a fellow Scout a simple first-aid skill is a great way to practice and gain mastery of the skill and will also allow you to complete requirement 7.

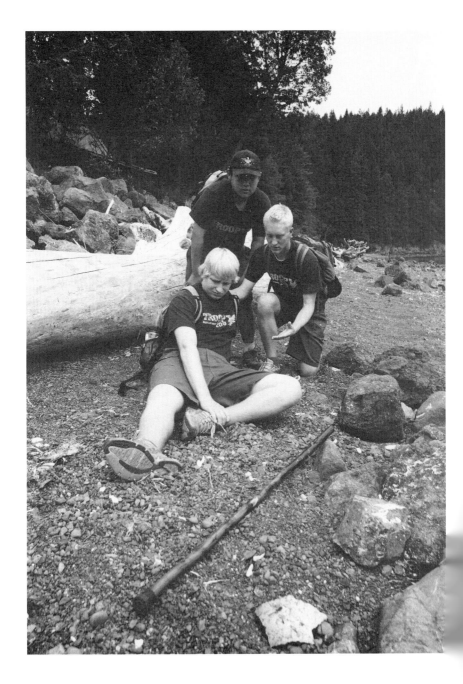

How to Handle an Emergency

Even the best plans can fall apart. Accidents will happen. People will become sick. You might be the person who is most able to take charge of an emergency scene. Here is how you should proceed.

Do Your Best

Good Samaritan laws legally protect anyone making a good-faith effort to help the victim of an injury or illness. Whenever you are confronted with a first-aid emergency, use your skills to the best of your ability. No one expects you to have the knowledge of a physician. However, Scouting's history is filled with stories of Scouts who used their training to help others, sometimes even saving lives.

1. Check the Scene

The site of an accident can be confusing, especially when serious injuries have occurred or there is more than one person involved. There are a number of things to consider. The hazard that caused the accident may still pose a threat. Seeing blood, broken bones, vomit, or people in pain might disturb bystanders and first-aiders.

Before you take any action, stop for a moment to look over the entire scene and collect your thoughts. Consider the following questions:

- What caused the accident?
- Are there dangers in the area?
- How many victims are there?
- If there are other people nearby, can they assist with first aid or with getting help?
- Will bystanders need guidance so that they do not become injured or ill themselves?

2. Call for Help

Should you encounter a situation where someone has more than a minor illness or injury, act quickly to get emergency medical help. You can reach emergency services in much of the United States by calling 911. Some communities use other emergency-alert systems such as dialing 0 or calling a local sheriff's office or fire department. Instruct a bystander or another first-aider to call for help immediately: *"You, call for help right now. Tell them where we are and what has happened, then report back to me."*

A wilderness camping trip can take you far from telephones. An injured Scout who can walk on his own or with some support may be able to hike to a road. A group of Scouts may be able to build a stretcher and carry a victim. For serious injuries, though, it is usually best to treat the victim at the accident site—provided that doing so would not further endanger the victim or the first-aiders—and send two or more people for help.

Mobile phones are unreliable in wilderness areas. If you take a mobile phone on an outing, have a backup plan for summoning emergency assistance.

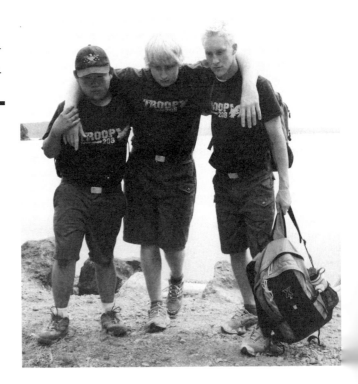

Write a note containing the following information and send it with the messengers:

- Location of the victim
- Description of the injuries or illness
- Time the injuries or illness occurred
- Treatment the victim has received
- Number of people with the victim and their general skill level for first aid
- Requests for special assistance or equipment, including food, shelter, or care for nonvictims

See "First-Aid Supplies and Skills" for information on how to build an improvised stretcher.

Activities on open water sometimes take people far from any help. Larger boats often have radio equipment that can be used to summon aid. When phones or radios are not available, however, passengers will need to make and carry out a plan for getting help. Such a plan might involve sending two people to the closest telephone to call for help.

In Case of Emergency

Many people carry mobile phones these days, but not everyone carries details of whom should be called on their behalf in case they are involved in a serious accident. If you add the acronym ICE—for "In Case of Emergency"—as a contact in your mobile phone, emergency workers can quickly find someone to notify about your condition. Ask your parent whom to list as your ICE contact.

3. Approach Safely

After assessing the situation and summoning help, determine the best way to reach the injured person or persons. Perhaps an accident victim is lying on a busy highway or has fallen and tumbled partway down a mountainside. Will you also be in danger if you dash onto the highway or rush down the slope? Figure out a safe way to approach the victim or to remove the dangers from an area. *Do not become an accident victim yourself.*

When a person is unconscious, assume it is OK to render aid.

Once you have figured out the safest way to approach, introduce yourself to injured persons and to bystanders. Assure them that medical professionals have been called and are on the way. Speaking in a calm voice, explain that you are a Scout trained in first aid and that you are there to help. Ask victims if they will allow you to assist them. Continue to speak to injured or ill persons as you administer first aid, keeping them informed of what you are doing.

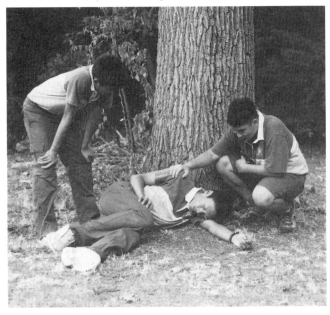

See "First-Aid Supplies and Skills" for precautions to be taken when moving accident victims.

Sometimes a victim's location threatens his or her safety and that of first-aiders. For example, suppose you are out hiking and a buddy falls into a stream or gets hurt while on an unstable boulder field or avalanche slope. It might be necessary to move him to a safer location before first-aid treatment can begin. To move him, get the help of several others in your group and lift the victim in the same position in which he was found. Then carry him to safety and gently put him down. (See "Moving an Ill or Injured Person" later in this pamphlet.) Take special care to prevent his neck from moving by supporting his head before, during, and after the emergency move.

Triage

Emergency situations involving more than one victim can require *triage* (pronounced *tree-ahge*)—quickly checking each victim for injuries or symptoms of illness and then determining how best to use available first-aid resources. In its simplest form, triage occurs whenever first-aiders approach an emergency scene that involves two or more persons who are injured or ill. Once on the scene, medical professionals will determine who requires urgent care, who can be treated later, who needs to be monitored in case his or her condition changes, and who is well enough to help out.

4. Provide Urgent Treatment

Breathing and *bleeding*—these are your immediate concerns when treating the victim of an accident or illness. Victims who have stopped breathing or who are bleeding severely are called *hurry cases* because their lives are in immediate danger. They require smart, timely action on the part of a first-aider.

Whenever you come upon an injured person, take no more than 15 to 20 seconds to do a quick survey of his or her condition to find out the following:

- *Is the person conscious and breathing?* If he or she seems to be unconscious, tap the person on the shoulder and ask (or shout) if he or she is all right. If the person does not respond, open the airway by tilting the head and lifting up on the chin, then place your ear near the mouth and nose where you can hear and feel the movement of air. Watch for the chest to rise and fall.

- *Is there severe bleeding?* Open rain gear and outer clothing that might hide wounds from view.

- *Are there other contributing factors?* Look for a medical ID bracelet, necklace, or card that might give information about allergies, diabetes, or other possible causes of an emergency situation. Persons who have asthma or allergies to insect stings or certain foods (such as peanuts) might carry treatment for their condition.

See "Life-Threatening Emergencies" for more details.

If the person is breathing, the breaths should not be irregular or shallow or short; the person should not be gasping for air.

For children age 11 and under, check for a pulse to make sure the heart is beating. This should not take more than 10 seconds.

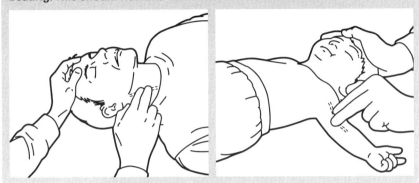

5. Protect From Further Injury

An important part of first aid is protecting an accident victim from further injury. Follow these guidelines.

- Avoid moving an injured person unless his or her body position makes it impossible to perform urgent first aid or he or she is in a dangerous location. If a person's position must be adjusted, for example, to allow them to breathe, do so with the minimum amount of movement.

- Stabilize the victim's head and neck to prevent any neck bones that may be broken from damaging the spinal cord. Ask a fellow first-aider or a bystander to hold the victim's head and neck steady to keep the neck in proper alignment.

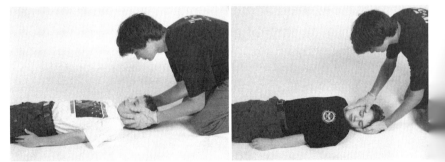

While awaiting emergency personnel, support the victim's head in the position you found it, in line with the person's body.

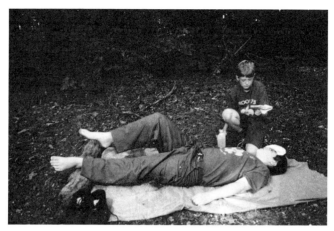

6. Treat Every Accident Victim for Shock

The circulatory system of a person who is injured or under great stress might not provide enough blood and oxygen to the tissues of the body. This condition is called *shock*, and it can be deadly (as organs can begin to fail). A shock victim can have some, all, or none of the following symptoms:

- Restlessness or irritability
- A feeling of weakness
- Confusion, fear, dizziness
- Skin that is moist, clammy, cool, and pale
- A quick, weak pulse
- Shallow, rapid, and irregular breathing
- Nausea and vomiting
- Extreme thirst

Serious injuries and sudden illnesses are almost always accompanied by some degree of shock, but the victim might not be affected right away. Treat every accident victim for shock even if no symptoms appear. Prompt first aid may prevent shock from setting in.

Fear and uncertainty can increase shock. In a calm voice, assure the person that everything possible is being done and that help is on the way. A person who appears to be unconscious may still be able to hear you. Never leave an accident victim alone unless you must briefly go to call for help.

First Aid for Shock

1. Try to eliminate the causes of shock by restoring breathing and circulation, controlling bleeding, relieving severe pain, and treating wounds.

2. Summon emergency aid.

3. Monitor the victim closely to make sure the airway stays open for breathing.

4. If the victim is not already doing so, help the injured person lie down. If you do not suspect back, neck, or head injuries, or fractures in the hip or leg, raise the feet about 12 inches to move blood from the legs to the vital organs.

5. Keep the victim warm with blankets, coats, or sleeping bags.

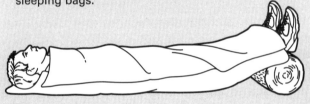

7. Make a Thorough Examination

By the time you have dealt with urgent conditions and provided treatment for shock, medical professionals are likely to have arrived. When their arrival is delayed or the location will require greater travel time, conduct a more thorough examination to be sure you have found all the victim's injuries that require attention. If the victim is alert, ask where it is painful and whether the victim can move the arms, legs, and so on. Get beneath jackets and other clothing that could obscure or hide wounds that are bleeding.

8. Plan a Course of Action

After conducting the examination, determine what to do next. The best course of action in most cases is to make the victim comfortable and continue to wait for medical help to arrive. Maintain treatment for shock, keep the airway open, monitor the victim for any changes, and be ready to provide any other treatment the victim might require.

In the backcountry it may be wise to set up camp and to shelter the victim with a tent. Rather than lifting a badly injured person into a tent, you can slit the floor of a standing tent and then place the tent over the person.

Be aware of your own needs, too, and those of others around you. Stay warm and dry. If a first-aid emergency lasts very long, be sure to eat and drink enough. Be aware that other group members may be frightened or disoriented by what they have seen. Be sure they do not wander off. Giving people specific responsibilities—fixing a meal or making camp, for example—can focus their attention and help keep them calm.

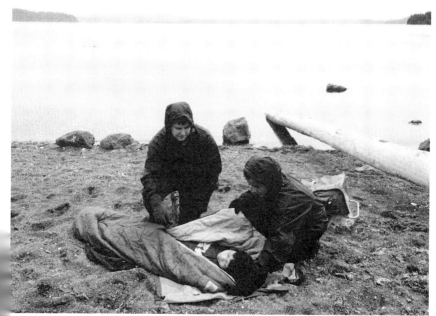

Learn all the first aid you can and review it often. Perhaps one day you will be able to do just the right thing at a time when your actions make all the difference.

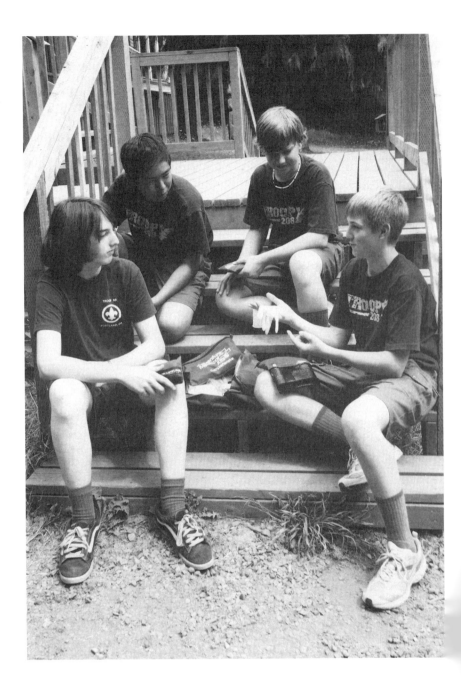

First-Aid Supplies and Skills

You cannot render first aid if you do not have the tools and supplies necessary to treat an injured or ill person. A well-stocked first-aid kit is an essential item for all first-aiders. Equally important is learning and practicing difficult first-aid skills such as how to safely transport an ill person or an accident victim.

Personal First-Aid Kit

Carrying a few first-aid items on hikes and campouts will allow you to treat scratches, blisters, and other minor injuries and to provide initial care for more serious emergencies. You should be able to fit everything in a resealable plastic bag. Always take your personal first-aid kit when you set out on a Scout adventure. Your kit should include as a minimum the following:

- ❏ Adhesive bandages (6)
- ❏ Sterile gauze pads, 3-by-3-inch (2)
- ❏ Adhesive tape (1 small roll)
- ❏ Moleskin, 3-by-6-inch (1)
- ❏ Soap (1 small bar) or alcohol-based hand sanitizing gel (1 travel size bottle)
- ❏ Triple antibiotic ointment (1 small tube)
- ❏ Scissors (1 pair)
- ❏ Nonlatex disposable gloves (1 pair)
- ❏ CPR breathing barrier (1)
- ❏ Pencil and paper

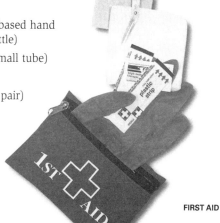

Home or Patrol/Troop First-Aid Kit

A more comprehensive first-aid kit suitable for home use or use by your patrol or troop can treat a wide range of injuries. After assembling your home kit, be sure everyone in your family knows where the kit is being stored. It also is a good idea to carry a first-aid kit in the car in case of roadside emergencies. On Scout outings, the patrol or troop first-aid kit can be carried in a fanny pack that is marked so that it will be easy for anyone to locate. At a minimum, the kit should contain the following:

❏ Roller bandage, 2-inch (1)

❏ Roller bandage, 1-inch (2)

❏ Adhesive tape, 1-inch (1 roll)

❏ Alcohol swabs (24)

❏ Assorted adhesive bandages (1 box)

❏ Elastic bandages, 3-inch-wide (2)

❏ Sterile gauze pads, 3-by-3-inch (12)

❏ Moleskin, 3-by-6-inch (4)

❏ Gel pads for blisters and burns (2 packets)

❏ Triple antibiotic ointment (1 tube)

❏ Triangular bandages (4)

❏ Soap (1 small bar) or alcohol-based hand sanitizing gel (1 travel size bottle)

❏ Scissors (1 pair)

❏ Tweezers (1 pair)

❏ Safety pins (12)

❏ Nonlatex disposable gloves (6 pairs)

❏ Protective goggles/safety glasses (1 pair)

❏ CPR breathing barrier (1)

❏ Pencil and paper

Moving an Ill or Injured Person

The decision to move an accident victim should be made carefully. In many cases, there will be emergency medical crews, fire department personnel, or others with special equipment and training who will transport an injured person. If, however, someone is in danger from fire, smoke, water, electrical hazards, poisonous gases, exposure, or other immediate danger, you must move that person to safety. You might also need to move an injured person in order to give that person proper care, or reach another victim. Move the person only as far as is necessary, and do not endanger yourself.

Sometimes you will find that a victim's injuries are minor enough that the person can move with some assistance. Before attempting to move someone, make sure the person is not suffering from any of the following conditions. Then determine the best technique to use for moving the victim or whether the victim should not be moved at all.

- Shock
- Heart attack
- Head, neck, or back (spinal) injury
- Frostbitten or burned feet
- Bone or joint injury at the hips or below

For a victim of a venomous bite or sting, getting the victim to medical attention is the most important goal. This may call for moving the victim before the swelling becomes too severe.

Here are some additional assists and hand carries to consider. Some can be performed by a single rescuer, while others require two or more rescuers. Practice single- and multiple-rescuer assists first with an uninjured person. This will help you work smoothly and safely during a real emergency.

> *Signals* includes both signs (what you would observe) as well as symptoms (what a person would communicate to you).

Single-Rescuer Assists

When an injured person must be moved, choose the method carefully to avoid making the injuries worse and to avoid injuring yourself. Recommended assists for a single rescuer include the following.

Walking assist. If the victim is conscious, has only minor injuries, and can move, you can safely help the person walk. Put one of the victim's arms around your neck. Hold that hand. Place your other arm around the person's waist.

Ankle drag. The fastest method for a short distance on a smooth surface, or to move someone who is too large or heavy to transport in any other way, is to drag the person by both ankles.

Shoulder drag.

For short distances over a rougher surface, and to move a conscious or unconscious person who may have head, neck, or back injuries, use the clothes drag. Firmly grab the person's clothing behind the shoulder and neck area and pull headfirst.

Blanket drag. Roll the person onto a blanket, coat, tarp, or tablecloth, cover the person as shown, if possible, and drag from behind the head.

One-person lift. You may be able to carry a child or someone who does not weigh much if you place one arm under the victim's knees and one around the upper back. Do not use this method if you suspect spinal injury.

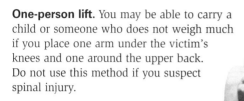

Firefighter carry. To travel longer distances, carry the victim over your shoulder if injuries will allow it. The firefighter carry should never be used if you suspect the victim has spinal injury.

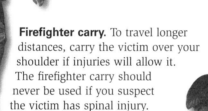

Pack-strap carry. The pack-strap carry is better for longer distances than the one-person lift and when the firefighter carry is not practical. Use this method only if you do not suspect spinal injury.

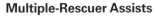

Multiple-Rescuer Assists

Recommended assists for two or more rescuers include the following.

Helping the person walk. If the victim is conscious and shows no signals of the conditions or injuries listed earlier, two rescuers can safely help the person walk. Put one of the victim's arms around each rescuer's neck. Hold the hands. Rescuers place their free arms around the victim's waist.

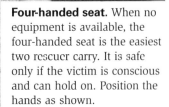

Four-handed seat. When no equipment is available, the four-handed seat is the easiest two rescuer carry. It is safe only if the victim is conscious and can hold on. Position the hands as shown.

Two-handed seat. Use this method if the victim is conscious but not seriously injured. Rescuers place arms on each other's shoulder and lock arms for stability as the victim gets into position, then move arms from shoulders to across the victim's back.

Chair carry. This is a good method for carrying an injured person up stairs or through narrow, winding spaces.

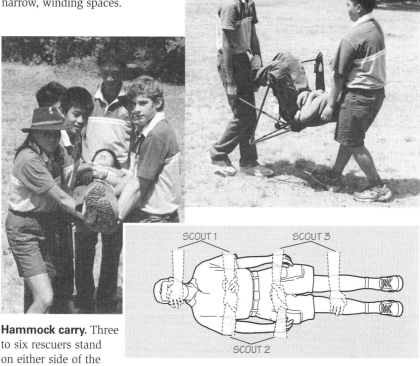

Hammock carry. Three to six rescuers stand on either side of the victim and link hands beneath the person.

Rescue From a Smoke-Filled Room

A smoke-filled room is an extremely hazardous environment. Rushing into a smoke-filled room or other dangerous scene to help someone will do no good if you also become a victim. If your safety will be threatened, wait until trained rescuers arrive.

Moving an injured or unconscious person should be done quickly. Avoid using any method that might make the victim's injuries worse. A victim can be moved to safety with any of the rescuer assists described in this chapter.

Stretchers

When a person must be moved for some distance or his or her injuries are serious, you should carry the person on a stretcher.

When available, use a litter or rescue basket made especially for transporting injured persons. If none is available, make one of the following improvised stretchers and use the method shown in the illustrations to place the victim on the improvised stretcher:

OVERLAP BOTTOMS OF THE SHIRTS.

Shirt stretcher. Make a stretcher out of two poles (longer than the victim is tall), for example, strong branches, tool handles, oars, or the poles from a wall tent. Secure two Scout shirts (inside out, with all the buttons buttoned) over the poles to form a stretcher. If possible, overlap the bottoms of the shirts to form a more secure bedding.

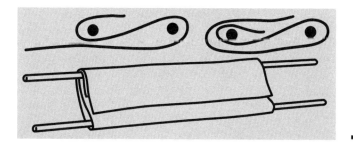

Blanket stretcher. Place a pole on the blanket. Fold over two-fifths of the blanket. Place a second pole 6 inches from the edge of the folded-over part. Bring the edge of the blanket over the pole. Fold over the rest of the blanket. The person's weight will keep the blanket from unwinding.

Board stretcher. Use a surfboard, door, bench, or ironing board to make this stretcher. A board stretcher is sturdier than a blanket stretcher but heavier and less comfortable for the victim. When two rescuers carry a stretcher, have one or two other rescuers, if available, walk at the sides to share the weight and help keep the victim from rolling off.

Transporting someone by stretcher (or improvised stretcher) can be difficult and exhausting work, requiring at least four rescuers. Stretcher bearers should trade off with each other to conserve their strength. At least one first-aider should stay by the victim's head at all times to monitor the person's condition and note any changes.

To place someone on a stretcher or improvised stretcher, have three rescuers hold the victim straight and steady. A fourth rescuer can slide the stretcher beneath the victim. Gently place the victim on the stretcher. The rescuers can lift and carry the stretcher.

If only three rescuers are available, they may try the hammock carry without a stretcher. First, they should position themselves at the victim's shoulders, torso, and legs to achieve full support. Then, they should lift and carry the victim, being sure to support the head, arms, and legs.

A stretcher can be formed by lashing three metal pack frames together. To work well, the frames must have roughly the same width. Use sleeping bags for padding.

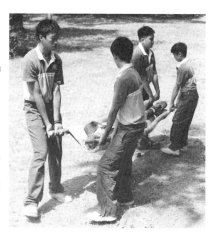

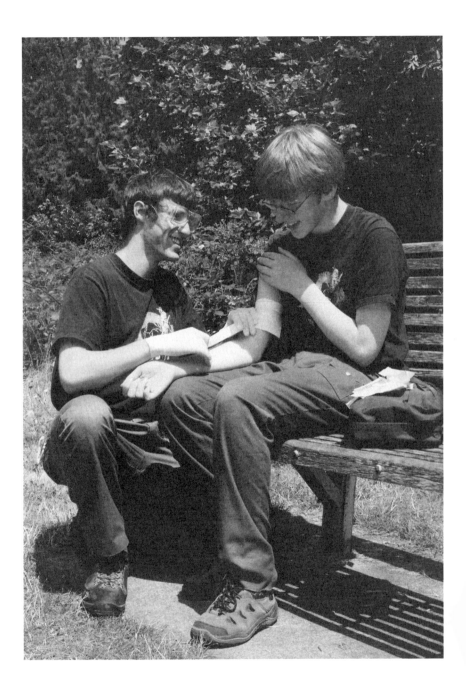

Minor Wounds and Injuries

Although you should be prepared to deal with a wide range of medical emergencies, your first-aid skills will probably be put to use most often in the treatment of relatively minor wounds and injuries.

Bruises

The black-and-blue mark that is typical of a bruise is caused by blood leaking into skin tissues, often as a result of a blow from a blunt object. The skin is not broken. Some bruises are indicators of more serious injuries including fractured bones or damage to internal organs. This type of bruise requires the attention of a physician.

Most bruises, however, can be treated by a person trained in first aid. To treat a bruise, place some ice (preferably) or a refreezable gel pack in a plastic bag or damp cloth. Place a towel or clean cloth over the bruised area and apply the ice pack for periods of no more than 20 minutes. This treatment will slow blood from leaking into the tissues. Minimizing movement of the affected area also slows bleeding into the bruise.

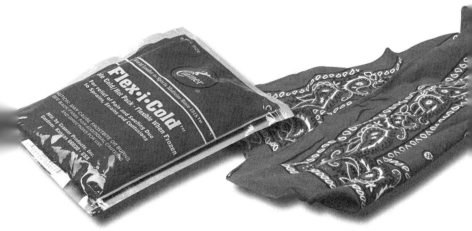

Puncture Wounds

Puncture wounds can be caused by pins, splinters, nails, or fishhooks. All can be dangerous because the nature of a puncture wound makes it hard to clean and easily infected. To treat a puncture wound, help flush out dirt or particles that may have been forced inside the wound when the injury occurred by irrigating the area with clean, running water for about five minutes. Use sterilized tweezers to pull out splinters, bits of glass, or other small objects you can see. If a large object is embedded, do not try to remove it. Control any bleeding, and stabilize the object with rolled or folded sterile gauze pads, apply a sterile bandage, and get the victim to a doctor.

Fishhook in the Skin

A fishhook embedded in the skin is a frequent outdoor injury. Remember two things: Do not try to remove a fishhook from the face or from an eye or an earlobe, and never try to remove an embedded hook by pulling it back the way it went in. Cut the fishing line and, if possible, let a doctor remove the hook from the flesh. If that isn't possible, you might have to do the job yourself. First, wash your hands with soap and warm water. Wear nonlatex disposable gloves and protective eyewear to avoid contact with blood.

Step 1—Wrap a 3-foot length of fishing line around the bend of the hook, as shown, and securely wrap the ends around your index or middle finger.

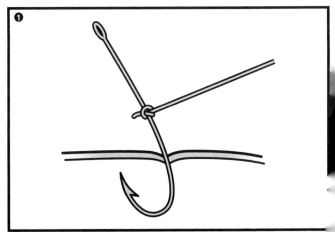

To sterilize tweezers, soak them in rubbing alcohol for a few minutes, or hold them over a flame for a few seconds, or place them in boiling water for a few minutes; cool before using.

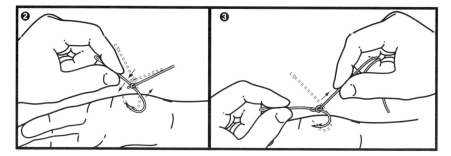

Step 2—Keep the affected body part flat and stable, then gently push down on the shank to free the barb from the injured tissue. The shank should be parallel to the injured tissue.

Step 3—Keep bystanders well away from the area. Give the line a quick, sharp jerk, and be careful to avoid getting snagged by the outcoming hook.

Step 4—Wash and bandage the injury, and keep the wound clean. Apply triple antibiotic ointment if there are no known allergies or sensitivities to the medication. See a doctor as soon as possible, because the risk of infection is high with this type of injury.

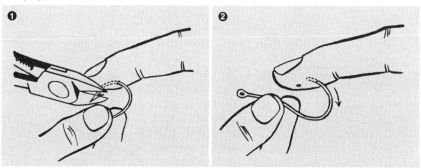

If the hook has lodged so that the barb is visible above the skin, try this method:

1. **Cut off the barbed end with wire cutters or pliers.**
2. **Back the shank of the hook out through the entry wound.**

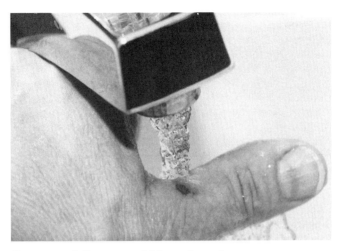

Cuts and Scrapes (Abrasions)

Cuts may be caused by knives, razors, or broken glass. An abrasion is a wound that occurs as a result of the outer layers of the skin being rubbed or scraped off. Abrasions may happen when the skin is scraped against a hard surface, for example, when a bicyclist falls onto the pavement. The wound may not bleed very much. The greatest danger lies in contamination and possible infection of the wound.

To protect yourself from cuts and scrapes, dress appropriately for the activity—for instance, jeans, boots, gloves, long-sleeved shirt. A few simple precautions can help you avoid the pain of the treatment and healing process.

Treat a minor cut or scrape by flushing the area with clean water for at least five minutes, or until all foreign matter appears to be washed away. Apply triple antibiotic ointment if the person has no known allergies or sensitivities to the medication, and then cover with a dry, sterile dressing and bandage or with an adhesive bandage.

When the weather is cold, keep the victim's hands and feet covered with mittens or socks. Remove mittens or socks frequently to check that circulation is not being restricted.

Dressings and Bandages

After cleaning a wound in which the skin has been broken, protect it with a dressing. A dressing is a protective covering placed over a wound that helps to control bleeding and absorb blood and wound secretions. Sterile dressings are free from germs and should be used to dress wounds whenever possible. If a sterile dressing is not available, use the cleanest cloth you have.

A bandage is a strip of material used to hold a dressing or splint in place. It helps immobilize, support, and protect the injury. Common bandages include rolls of gauze, elastic bandages, and triangular bandages. Combination dressing-bandages include adhesive strips with attached gauze pads.

Secure the dressing with a bandage or tape. Watch for swelling, color changes, or coldness of the fingertips or toes. If any of these symptoms appear, it is a signal that circulation is being compromised. Loosen bandages if the victim complains of tingling or numbness.

When using a bandage to secure a dressing, be sure not to wrap it too tightly. Be sure the person's fingertips or toes are accessible when a splint or bandage is applied to the arm or leg.

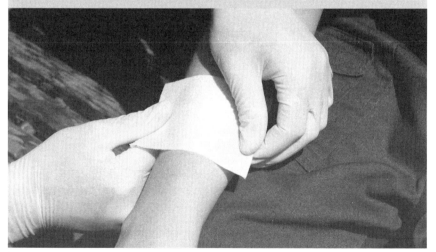

To dress and bandage a wound, use a dressing large enough to extend an inch or more beyond the edge of the wound. Hold the dressing over the wound and lower it directly into place. If the dressing slips onto the surrounding skin before it has been anchored, discard it and use a fresh dressing.

Blisters on the Hand and Foot

Blisters are pockets of fluid that form when the skin is aggravated by friction. Foot blisters are common injuries among backpackers, whereas blisters on the hands might be more common among canoeists. To help prevent foot blisters, wear shoes or boots that fit, change socks if they become sweaty or wet, and pay attention to how your feet feel. To help prevent blisters on the hands, wear gloves for protection and pay attention to how your hands feel.

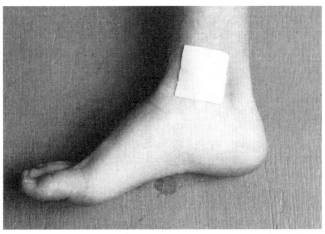

Blisters are best left unbroken. If a blister does break, treat the broken blister as you would a minor cut or abrasion. Diabetics who develop blisters should see a physician.

A *hot spot*—the tender area as a blister starts to form—is a signal to stop immediately. To treat a hot spot or blister, cover the pinkish, tender area with a piece of moleskin or molefoam slightly larger than the hot spot. Use several layers if necessary. There are a couple of helpful new products on the market— Second Skin® and Blist-O-Ban®—that may be worth trying. Follow the manufacturer's instructions. Change bandages every day to help keep wounds clean and avoid infection.

If you must continue your activity even though you think a small blister will burst, you might want to drain the fluid. First, wash the skin with soap and water, then sterilize a pin in the flame of a match. Prick the blister near its lower edge and press out the fluid. Keep the wound clean with a sterile bandage or gel pad and moleskin.

Protection From Bloodborne Pathogens

Whenever you provide first-aid care—no matter how minor the wound or injury—you should take steps to protect yourself and others from bloodborne pathogens, viruses, or bacteria carried in the blood that can cause disease in humans and may be present in the blood or other body fluids of the victims you treat. Bloodborne pathogens include the human immunodeficiency virus (HIV), which causes AIDS, and the hepatitis B and C viruses, which cause liver disease.

Recommendations from the Boy Scouts of America:

• Treat all blood as if it were contaminated with bloodborne pathogens.

• Thoroughly wash your hands with soap and warm water before and after treating a sick or injured person.

• Never use your bare hands to stop bleeding. Use a protective barrier, preferably nonlatex disposable gloves (a new, unused plastic food storage bag will work in a pinch).

In some situations, such as a life-threatening one, it might not be possible or practical to spend 15 or 20 seconds washing your hands. Do the best you can, and use your good judgment.

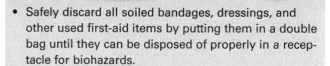

• Safely discard all soiled bandages, dressings, and other used first-aid items by putting them in a double bag until they can be disposed of properly in a receptacle for biohazards.

• Always wash your hands and other exposed skin with soap and warm water or an alcohol-based hand sanitizer immediately after treating a victim, even if protective equipment was used.

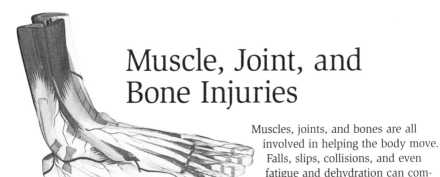

Muscle, Joint, and Bone Injuries

Muscles, joints, and bones are all involved in helping the body move. Falls, slips, collisions, and even fatigue and dehydration can compromise or injure these body parts.

Muscle Cramps

Muscle cramps most often affect the legs, but they also can occur in the muscles of the ribs, arms, and hands.

A muscle cramp occurs when a muscle contracts on its own and does not easily relax. They tend to happen most when the body is fatigued and the muscles have not been stretched well. Dehydration, exertion in hot weather, and depletion of electrolytes (calcium, chloride, phosphate, potassium, sodium) in the body may also lead to muscle cramping. With severe cramping, the muscle may feel hard and knotted.

Allow a person experiencing muscle cramps to rest. Often a cramp will disappear on its own in a few minutes. To help recovery, gently massage the muscle and lightly stretch it. If the weather is warm and the person has been exercising, be sure the person rehydrates with water or, ideally, a sports drink that will help the body and restore its proper electrolyte balance.

Decrease the likelihood of muscle cramps by staying in good physical shape, stretching before exercising, warming down, and drinking plenty of fluids before, during, and after you work out.

Sprains and Strains

A *sprain* occurs when an ankle, wrist, or other joint is bent far enough to overstretch the ligaments, the tough bands that hold joints together. Twisting an ankle while running is one way a person could sustain a sprain. A *strain* occurs when muscles are overstretched, creating tears in the muscle fibers. Lower back pain is often the result of muscles strained by overuse or by lifting loads that are too heavy.

Minor sprains and strains cause only mild discomfort, but more serious sprains and strains might be temporarily disabling. A sprained joint will be tender and painful when moved and might show swelling and discoloration. Strained backs, arms, and legs will also be tender and can hurt if activity continues.

Assume that any injury to a joint also may include a bone fracture. Use the following procedure to treat sprains and strains and prevent further injury. Have the victim take any weight off of the injured joint and instruct the person not to use the joint. Do not try to move or straighten an injured limb. Cover any open wounds with a sterile dressing. Apply ice packs or cold compresses to the affected area for no more than 20 minutes at a time. Be sure to place a barrier such as a thin towel between the ice pack and bare skin. Seek medical treatment if the pain is persistent or severe.

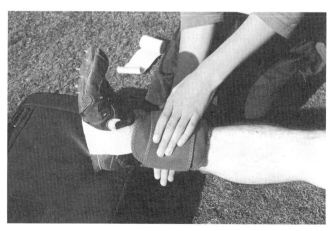

If continued icing is needed, remove the pack for 20 minutes before reapplying.

Sprains While Hiking

If someone suffers an ankle sprain during a hike and your group must keep walking, do not remove the hiking boot from the injured foot. The boot will help support the ankle. If you do take the boot off, the injury may swell so much it will not be possible to get the boot back on. Reinforce the ankle by wrapping it, boot and all, with a bandage, neckerchief, or some other strip of cloth.

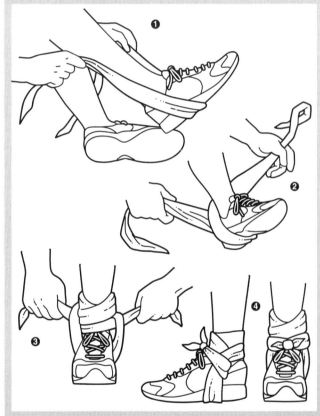

As soon as you have reached your destination, have the person take off the boot. Treat with cold packs and seek medical care.

Broken Bones

A fall, a violent blow, a collision—all these can cause a *fracture*, or broken bone. When you suspect a fracture, do not move the person. Look for abnormal shape or position of a bone or joint, and swelling or a bluish color at the injured site.

Ask the victim these questions:

• Did you hear or feel a bone snap?

• Do you feel pain when you press on the skin over the suspected fracture?

• Are you unable to move the injured limb?

If the victim answers "yes" to these questions, the person likely has a fracture.

> Before administering first aid, you should try to obtain the victim's consent. If the victim is unconscious, disoriented, or otherwise appears unable to knowingly grant consent, you can assume it is all right to proceed.

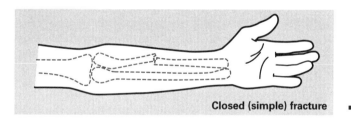

Closed (simple) fracture

Closed (Simple) Fracture. A *closed fracture* (also known as a *simple fracture*) is a broken bone that does not cut through the skin. For a closed fracture, do the following.

• Call 911 or your local emergency-response number.

• Treat hurry cases—no signs of life (movement and breathing) in adults; in children and infants, no signs of life and no pulse.

• Protect the spinal column by supporting the victim's head and neck in the position found.

• Treat for shock (but avoid raising a leg that might be broken).

See "Life-Threatening Emergencies" for procedures to follow in hurry cases.

Do not try to
replace nor move
a bone that seems
to be sticking out
from the wound.

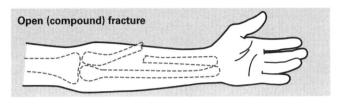

Open (compound) fracture

Open (Compound) Fracture. An *open fracture* (also known as a *compound fracture*) is a broken bone that breaks through the skin and creates an open wound. Take the following actions for an open fracture.

- Call 911 or your local emergency-response number.
- Treat hurry cases—no signs of life (movement and breathing) in adults; in children and infants, no signs of life and no pulse.
- Protect the spinal column by supporting the victim's head and neck in the position found.
- Control bleeding by placing a sterile gauze around the wound as you would for an embedded object. Do not use direct pressure, as that could move the bone.
- Do not try to clean the wound.
- Treat for shock (but avoid raising a leg that might be broken).

Whether you are treating a closed or an open fracture, allow the person to lie where you found him or her, unless the site poses an immediate hazard to the victim or rescuers. Make the person comfortable by tucking blankets, sleeping bags, or clothing under and over the body.

The saying "splint
it where it lies"
is usually
good advice.

SPLINTS

If the victim must be moved, splinting a broken bone can help relieve pain and reduce the chances of additional injury. A splint is any material, soft or rigid, that can be bound to a fractured limb. Use splinting only if necessary, to stabilize the injured area and prevent it from moving and causing further injury and pain. Make the splint long enough to immobilize the joints above, below, and on either side of a fracture, as needed.

Make splints from whatever is handy—boards, branches, blankets, hiking sticks, ski poles, shovel handles, or tent-pole sections. Folded newspapers, magazines, or pieces of cardboard or a sleeping pad will work, too. Take enough time to design an effective splint and secure it with good knots to provide enough support.

Padding allows a splint to fit better and can make the victim more comfortable. Cushion a splint with clothing, blankets, pillows, crumpled paper, or other soft material. Hold the splints and padding in place with neckerchiefs, handkerchiefs, roller bandages, or other wide strips of cloth, as shown.

HOW TO SPLINT AN INJURED LIMB

Splint all fractures and suspected fractures in the same position as you found them. Do not try to straighten or reposition the injured area.

Step 1—Keep the area above and below the injury still and stable.

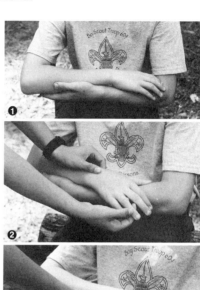

Step 2—Check for circulation (feeling, warmth, color).

Step 3—Extend splints beyond the joint above and the joint below the suspected injury. Minimize movement while applying splints by providing support above and below the fracture.

Step 4—Secure splints with bandages, neckerchiefs, or other wide strips of cloth. Tie at least one place above the injured area and one below. Do not tie bandages directly over the injury itself.

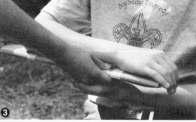

Step 5—After the splint is in place, recheck for circulation (feeling, warmth, color) to make sure you haven't cut off circulation.

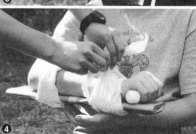

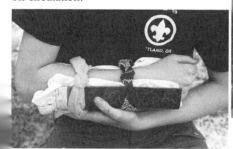

Improvised splint for the lower arm, using a magazine and padding

Soft splint on the lower leg. When applying a soft splint on the lower leg, do not remove the injured person's shoe; it will provide support and help control swelling.

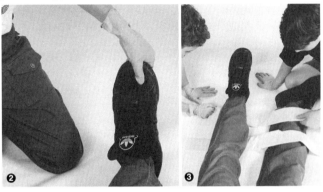

Step 1—Support the injured area, above and below, with one hand under the ankle and the other hand keeping the foot upright.

Step 2—Without removing the shoe, carefully check for circulation (feeling, warmth, color).

Step 3—Position several triangular bandages, as shown, under the injured area.

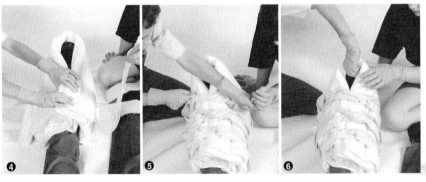

Step 4—Gently wrap something soft (small blanket or towel) around the injured area, as shown.

Step 5—Tie the triangular bandages in place securely with knots.

Step 6—Recheck the area for circulation (feeling, warmth, color). No circulation is an indication that the bandage is too tight and should be loosened.

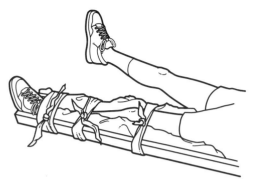

Lower-leg fracture. Use splints that are long enough to reach from the middle of the thigh to past the heel. Place one splint on each side of the injured limb and bind them together.

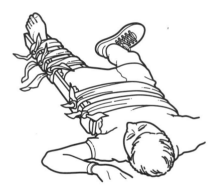

Upper-leg fracture. Apply two padded splints, one outside the leg extending from heel to armpit, the other inside the leg from the heel to the crotch. Bind the splints together.

The muscles of the upper leg are strong enough to pull the ends of a broken thigh bone into the flesh, sometimes causing serious internal bleeding that may pose a threat to the victim's life. For this reason, in addition to the first aid described here for a thigh bone (femur) fracture, treat this injury as a hurry case. Call for medical help immediately. Keep the victim still and quiet. Control any bleeding, and treat for shock.

SLINGS

Slings help support an injured hand, arm, collarbone, or shoulder.

Step 1—Support the injured limb above and below the injured area.

Step 2—Check the injured area for circulation (feeling, warmth, color).

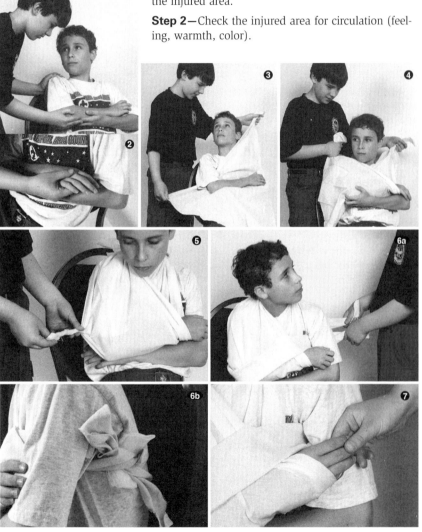

Step 3—Position a triangular sling (such as a folded Scout neckerchief or a large triangular bandage) across the chest as shown. If one is available, place a clean gauze bandage over the side of the neck for comfort, at the area where the sling will be knotted.

Step 4—Bring the upper free end of the sling behind the neck and the lower free corner upward (as shown) and tie the ends together with a square knot, forming the sling.

Step 5—To keep the injured area more stable, bind the sling to the chest using a second triangular bandage. Roll the bandage up as shown. Comfortably but not too loosely position the bandage above the injured area, over the sling and across the victim's front.

Step 6—Bring one end of the rolled-up bandage under the victim's uninjured arm and the other side around the back (6a). Tie the ends together with a square knot and put a clean gauze pad under the knot for comfort (6b).

Step 7—Recheck the injured area for feeling, warmth, and color.

Cravat Bandage

To make a cravat bandage from a Scout neckerchief or triangular bandage:

1. Fold the point up to the long edge.

2. Finish by folding the bottom edge several times toward the top edge.

3. Tie all bandages in place with square knots.

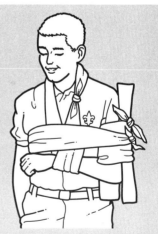

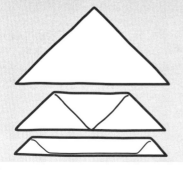

Upper-arm fracture. Tie a splint to the outside of the upper-arm. Place the arm in a sling with the hand raised about 3 inches above level, then use a cravat bandage to hold the upper arm against the side of the chest. The body will act as a splint to immobilize the elbow and shoulder.

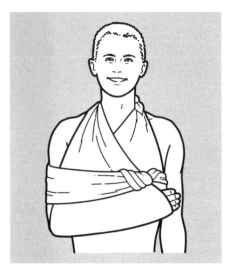

Collarbone or shoulder fracture. Place the forearm in a sling with the hand raised higher than the elbow, then tie the upper arm against the side of the body with a wide cravat bandage. No further splinting is necessary.

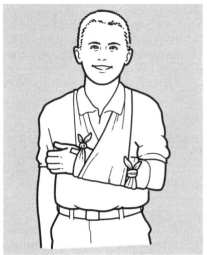

Lower-arm fracture. Splint to hold the hand and forearm motionless. Placing the splinted arm in a sling with the hand slightly raised will also immobilize the elbow joint.

Head, Neck, and Back Injuries

The backbone (spinal column) is made up of small bones called *vertebrae* that surround and protect the spinal cord. If a vertebra is broken or dislocated, the spinal cord may be injured. Fractures of the head, neck, and back are extremely dangerous, because movement might further damage the spinal cord and cause permanent paralysis or even death.

Whenever someone has fallen, been involved in an automobile accident, or suffered a blow to the head, assume there is an injury to the head, neck, or back. Such injuries are often not easy to detect. The victim may or may not be suffering from pain, paralysis, cuts and bruises, or swelling. The injured area may be deformed or abnormally shaped, or there may be no symptoms at all. Someone with a head injury might be disoriented, irritable, confused, or combative—symptoms that can be present right away or might develop over time. Always proceed with great caution when you are aiding a person whom you suspect has head, neck, or back injuries.

It is safe to suspect possible head, neck, or back injury when the victim

- Has been in a motor vehicle crash
- Has fallen from higher than a standing height
- Complains of neck or back pain
- Feels tingling or weakness in the fingers or toes
- Is not fully alert
- Appears to be intoxicated
- Appears to be frail or over 65 years of age

When you suspect an injury to the head, neck, or back, follow these steps.

Step 1—Stabilize the head and neck of the victim until it can be determined whether the spinal column has been injured. A first-aider or a bystander can hold the victim's head and neck steady.

Step 2—Provide urgent treatment if necessary.

Step 3—Do not move the person or let him or her move unless threatened by an immediate danger such as fire, potential avalanche, or highway traffic.

Step 4—If the victim is having trouble breathing, gently adjust the position of the head and neck just enough to maintain an open airway. Do not put a pillow under the head.

Step 5—Treat for shock but do not unnecessarily change the victim's position.

Whenever you suspect head, neck, or back injuries and the victim must be moved (to open an airway, for example, or to get the person out of the path of danger), ask other Scouts or bystanders to help so that the victim's body can be turned or lifted all at once without causing any twists or turns.

See "Life-Threatening Emergencies" for more information about urgent treatment. For more on moving an accident victim, see "First-Aid Supplies and Skills."

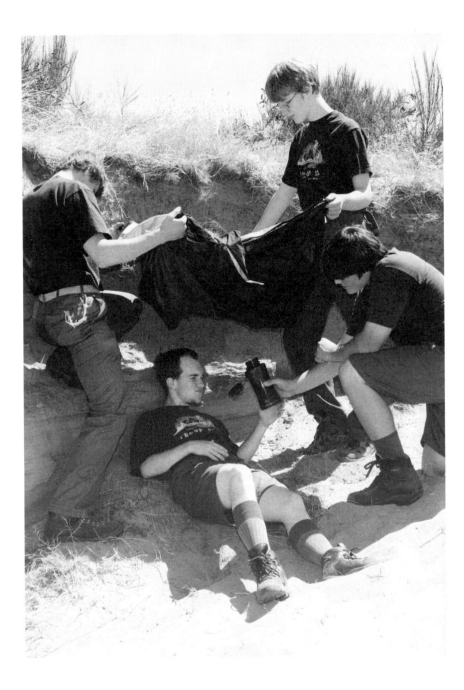

Cold- and Heat-Related Conditions and Injuries

The human body works best if it has a constant temperature of 98.6 degrees. A person who is exposed to cold environmental conditions and loses body heat faster than it can be generated will be in grave danger. The person's body temperature may become too low to support life. Likewise, a person whose body has overheated and cannot cool itself sufficiently may die if fast emergency medical care cannot be found. These temperature-related emergencies require fast, lifesaving first aid.

Hypothermia

Hypothermia occurs when a person's body is losing more heat than it can generate. It is a danger for anyone who is not dressed warmly enough, although exposure to cold is seldom the only cause. Dehydration is a common contributing factor to hypothermia. Wind, rain, hunger, and exhaustion can further compound the danger. Temperatures do not need to be below freezing, either. A hiker caught out in a cool, windy rain shower without proper rain gear can be at great risk. A swimmer too far out in chilly water or a paddler who capsizes also is at risk for hypothermia.

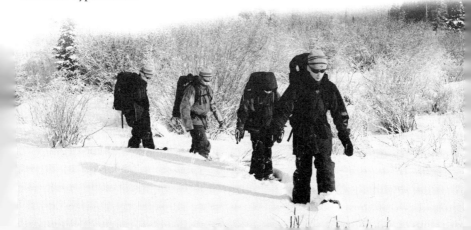

First Aid for Hypothermia

A hypothermia victim may experience numbness, fatigue, irritability, slurred speech, uncontrollable shivering, poor judgment or decision making, and loss of consciousness.

Treat a hypothermia victim by preventing the person from getting colder. After summoning help, use any or all of the following methods to help bring the body temperature back up to normal:

- If fully conscious and able to swallow, have the person drink warm liquids (soup, fruit juices, water; no caffeine or alcohol).

- Move the person into the shelter of a building or a tent. Remove wet clothing. Get him or her into dry, warm clothes or wrap the person in blankets, clothing, or anything handy that could be used, like jackets or a sleeping bag.

- Wrap towels around water bottles filled with warm fluid, then position the bottles in the armpit and groin areas.

- Monitor the person closely for any change in condition. Do not rewarm the person too quickly (for instance, by immersing the person in warm water); doing so can cause an irregular and dangerous heartbeat (rhythms).

If one person is being treated for hypothermia, the rest of a group might also be at risk. Protect yourselves by taking shelter, putting on layers of warm clothing, and having something to eat and something warm to drink.

Frostbite

Frostbite is a condition that occurs when skin is exposed to temperatures cold enough that ice crystals begin to form in the tissues. A frostbite victim might complain that the ears, nose, fingers, or feet feel painful and then numb, but sometimes the person will not notice any such sensation. Grayish-white patches on the skin—indicating that ice crystals have begun to form in the top layers of the skin—are signals of the first stage of frostbite, or *frostnip.* With continued exposure, frostnip worsens and the freezing extends to deeper layers of the skin and to the muscles. Frostbite can be very serious, as it can cut off blood flow to the affected area and lead to gangrene, or tissue death.

> Far from the warmth of the body's core, toes and fingers are especially vulnerable, as are the nose, ears, and cheeks.

Dehydration increases the danger of frostbite, so cold-weather travelers must be just as diligent about drinking fluids as they are when the weather is hot.

First Aid for Frostbite

If you suspect that frostbite extends below skin level, remove wet clothing and wrap the injured area in a dry blanket. Get the victim under the care of a physician as soon as possible. Do not massage the area or rub it with snow. **Rewarm the area only if there is no chance of refreezing.** Expose the affected area to warm (100 to 105 degrees) water until normal color returns and it feels warm, and bandage the area loosely (placing dry, sterile gauze between fingers and toes).

To treat frostnip, move the victim into a tent or building, then warm the injured area. If an ear or cheek is frozen, remove a glove and warm the injury with the palm of your hand. Slip a frostnipped hand under your clothing and tuck it beneath an armpit. Treat frostnipped toes by putting the victim's bare feet against the warm skin of your belly.

Dehydration

The human body is 70 percent water, which is essential to maintain our body temperature. Vital organs like the brain and the kidneys will not function well without enough water. We lose water mostly by breathing, sweating, digestion, and urination. When we lose more water than we take in, we become *dehydrated.* Symptoms of mild dehydration include increased thirst, dry lips, and dark yellow urine. Symptoms of moderate to severe dehydration include severe thirst, dry mouth with little saliva, dry skin, weakness, dizziness, confusion, nausea, fainting, muscle cramps, loss of appetite, decreased sweating (even with exertion), decreased urine production, and less frequent and dark brown urine.

The importance of drinking plenty of fluids cannot be overemphasized. Do not wait until you feel thirsty—thirst is an indication you are already becoming dehydrated.

First Aid for Dehydration

To treat mild dehydration, drink plenty of water or a sports drink to replace fluids and minerals. Drink one to two quarts (or liters) of liquids over two to four hours. See a physician for moderate or severe dehydration. Severe dehydration requires emergency care; the victim will need intravenous fluids. Rest for 24 hours and continue drinking fluids. Avoid tiring physical activity. Although most people begin to feel better within a few hours, it takes about 36 hours to completely restore the fluids lost in dehydration.

Heat Exhaustion

Heat exhaustion can be brought on by a combination of dehydration and a warm environment. Heat exhaustion is not uncommon during outdoor activities conducted in hot weather, especially if participants are not fully acclimated to the conditions. Symptoms of heat exhaustion include severe lack of energy, general weakness, headache, nausea, faintness, and sweating; cool, pale, moist skin; and a rapid pulse.

First Aid for Heat Exhaustion

Get the person in the shade (or an air-conditioned vehicle or building). Encourage him or her to drink small amounts of fluids, such as cool water or a sports drink. Apply water to the skin and clothing and fan the person to help the cooling process. Raising the legs may help prevent a feeling of faintness when the person stands. Usually after two or three hours of rest and fluids, the victim will feel better but should rest for the remainder of the day and be extra careful about staying hydrated.

Dehydration can play a significant role in a number of serious conditions, including heat exhaustion, heat-stroke, hypothermia, and frostbite. Dehydration can happen in hot- *and* cold-weather conditions.

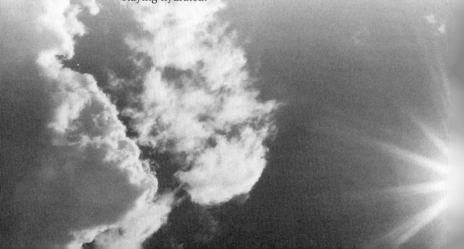

Heatstroke

Heatstroke—much more serious than heat exhaustion—can lead to death if not treated immediately. Left untreated, heat exhaustion can develop into heatstroke. In heatstroke, the body's cooling system begins to fail and the person's core temperature rises to life-threatening levels (above 105 degrees). One type of heatstroke develops in young, healthy people from dehydration and overexertion in hot weather, especially in high humidity. Symptoms of exercise-related heatstroke can include any symptoms of heat exhaustion as well as hot, sweaty, red skin, confusion, disorientation, and a rapid pulse.

The other type of heatstroke usually happens in elderly people when the weather is very hot, especially with high humidity. The symptoms are similar to exercise-related heatstroke except that the skin is hot *and* dry because there is no sweating.

First Aid for Heatstroke

Heatstroke is a life-threatening condition. Call for medical assistance immediately. While waiting for medical personnel to arrive, work to lower the victim's temperature. Move the person to an air-conditioned or shady area. Loosen tight clothing and further cool the victim by fanning and applying wet towels. If you have ice packs, wrap them in a thin barrier (such as a thin towel) and place them under the armpits and against the neck and groin. If the person is able to drink, give small amounts of cool water.

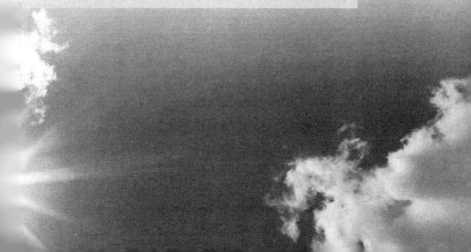

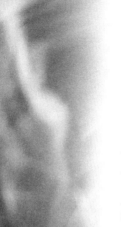

Burns

A spark from a campfire, boiling water spilled from a pot, a faulty wire, a mishap with chemicals in a science class, the rays of the sun on bare skin—the causes of burns are many. Burns are generally characterized by degree, or the severity of the skin and tissue damage.

Superficial (First-Degree) Burns

Mild burns, such as you might get from touching a baking dish that has just come out of an oven, will cause a painful reddening of the skin. Such burns are classified as *superficial,* or first-degree burns—they affect only the outer layer of skin, or *epidermis.* Treat them by holding the burn under cold water or applying cool, wet compresses until the pain eases. Superficial burns do not usually require further medical treatment unless they cover more than 20 to 25 percent of the body.

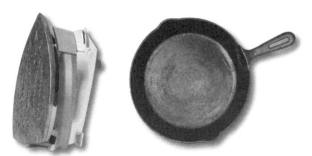

Remember to check the scene before you proceed. Always get a victim away from the source of a burn before proceeding with treatment.

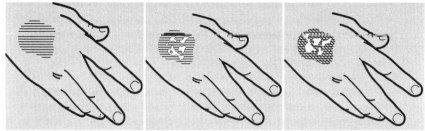

| Superficial | Partial thickness | Full thickness |

While the general public continues to be more familiar with the terms "first degree," "second degree," and "third degree" to classify burns, medical professionals identify burns by their "thickness." For instance, minor (first-degree) burns are called *superficial*. Those that cause blistering of the skin (second-degree) are called *partial-thickness* burns. The most serious burns (third-degree) are called *full-thickness* burns.

Partial-Thickness (Second-Degree) Burns

A *partial-thickness* (second-degree) burn affects the epidermis and part of the layer of skin below it, the *dermis*. Partial-thickness burns are more serious than superficial burns and typically include a reddening and blistering of the skin. Being scalded by boiling water is an example of an accident that could result in partial-thickness burns. To treat such burns, first remove the person from the source of the burn. Cool the burned area with cold, running water until the pain is relieved. Let the burn dry, then protect it with a loosely applied, sterile gauze pad and bandage.

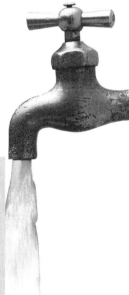

Get immediate medical treatment for the victim if the burns

- Cause trouble breathing
- Cover more than one body part or a large surface
- Have caused possible burns to the airway (such as burns to the mouth and nose)
- Affect the head, neck, hands, feet, or genitalia
- Are full thickness and the victim is younger than age 5 or older than age 60
- Are the result of chemicals, explosions, or electricity

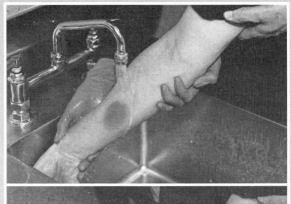

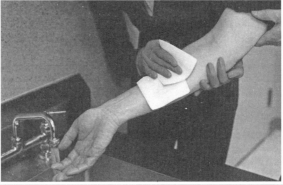

Treat thermal burns like this scalded forearm by running the affected area under cool running water, or by applying cool, wet compresses. Cover the area loosely with a sterile gauze pad and bandage.

Never break burn blisters. Doing so will create an open wound that may become infected. Do not apply butter, creams, ointments, or sprays—they are difficult to remove and may slow the healing process.

Full-Thickness (Third-Degree) Burns

Full-thickness (third-degree) burns are very serious. They destroy the epidermis and the dermis. A victim who has been exposed to open flames, electricity, or chemicals may sustain full-thickness burns. The skin may be burned away and the flesh charred. If nerves are damaged, the victim may feel no pain. Such burns constitute a medical emergency. Do not try to remove any clothing, as it may be sticking to the victim's flesh. After cooling the burn, cover the burned area with dry, sterile dressings, treat for shock, and seek immediate medical attention.

Chemical Burns

Chemical burns can be caused by exposure of the skin or eyes to substances that are strong acids or strong bases such as model glue, drain cleaners, toilet-bowl cleaners, metal cleaners, and battery acid.

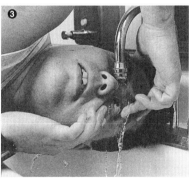

Here are steps for treating a chemical burn.

Step 1—Using gloves or a piece of cloth, brush off powdered chemicals from the victim's skin. Remove any of the victim's clothing with chemicals on it. Do not contaminate yourself in the process.

Step 2—Immediately flood the affected area with cool, clean water. Continue flushing the wound for at least 20 minutes to remove traces of the chemical.

Step 3—If the chemical got into the eyes, flush the eyes with clean water. It may be easier to have the victim lie down while flushing the eyes with water. Act as quickly as possible. Continue flushing for at least 15 minutes, or until emergency medical professionals arrive.

Step 4—Cover the burns loosely with sterile dressings or gauze.

Step 5—Get medical help by calling 911 or your local emergency-response number immediately. If you know the name of the product or substance that caused the burn, be sure to inform emergency workers.

The damage from a chemical burn can take hours—even days—to fully develop. For this reason, it is initially difficult to evaluate the extent of the burn. The most important first aid for a chemical burn is to dilute the exposure by continuously flushing the area with water for at least 15 to 20 minutes, or until emergency medical help arrives. Remember also that inhaling chemicals can damage your airway and lungs, too.

Burns From Dry Chemicals

As long as the dry chemical is on the skin, it will continue to burn. So, it's important to quickly brush off as much of the chemical as possible using a gloved hand. Then flush the area with tap water, taking care not to recontaminate the victim or to contaminate yourself.

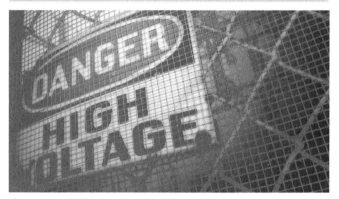

Electrical Burns

Never touch a person who is in contact with a live electrical power source.

If electricity travels through a part of your body, you can get an electrical burn. Besides a burn, too much electricity can even stop the heart from beating correctly or damage other internal organs. Superficial and partial-thickness burns from electricity look like burns from too much heat; the skin may look charred. Full-thickness electrical burns may not leave charred skin. Instead, the skin can look leathery and white and be hard to the touch. Call 911 or the local emergency-response number if someone has an electrical burn.

If you encounter a victim of an electrical burn, shut off the power at its source, and call an ambulance immediately. Check the scene for safety, then take the following steps:

Step 1—Perform rescue breathing or CPR if the victim is not breathing or moving. (See "Life-Threatening Emergencies.")

Step 2—Cover burns with sterile gauze pads. Cool electrical burns as for thermal burns.

Step 3—Treat for shock.

Sunburn

Sunburn is a common injury among people who enjoy being outdoors. Most sunburns are first-degree burns, but prolonged exposure to the sun can cause blistering—a second-degree burn. Repeated sunburns over a long period of time can cause skin damage and increase the risk of skin cancer. People with lighter skin are most at risk, although others are not immune.

Treat painful sunburn as for any heat burn or with cool, damp or wet cloths; change the cloths frequently. Prevent further injury by getting the person under shade. If no shade is available or you are out on a hiking or boating trip, have the person wear a brimmed hat, pants, and a long-sleeved shirt for protection from the sun.

It is best to prevent sunburn. Whenever you are outdoors, use plenty of sunscreen with a sun protection factor (SPF) rating of at least 15. Apply sunscreen liberally about a half-hour before sunlight exposure and reapply every two hours, especially if you are sweating or have been in water. A broad-brimmed hat, long-sleeved shirt, and long pants provide even more protection.

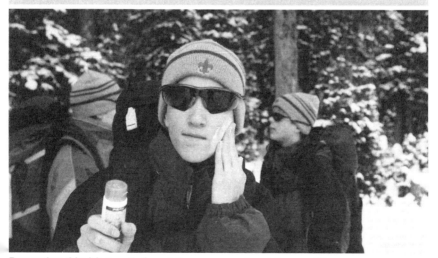

Remember this: It's easy to forget the sunscreen in wintry conditions.

Other First-Aid Cases

As a first-aider, you will encounter many relatively minor cases. Nevertheless, always take all injuries, illnesses, or conditions seriously. They can be symptoms of a more serious health threat. Abdominal pain, for example, could be among the first signals of appendicitis. A fainting spell could occur as a result of a heart attack, stroke, or internal bleeding.

Many people have heath conditions such as diabetes or epilepsy. Signals of these conditions can flare up unexpectedly and may require first aid. Whenever you prepare for a group outing such as a camping or canoeing trip, find out if any participants have such conditions and have them inform group leaders of their health histories, treatment regimens, medications, and the locations of those medications.

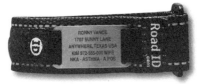

Any important medical information should be included on a medical ID bracelet.

Fainting

Sometimes fainting is a signal of a more serious condition such as an irregular heartbeat, heart valve problems, or internal bleeding.

Fainting is a brief loss of consciousness. It usually occurs because there is temporary loss of blood flow to the brain. It can be caused by getting up too quickly or standing too long, by overheating or dehydration, by emotional stress such as fright or bad news, or by severe pain.

Fainting can occur suddenly, or there might first be signals such as dizziness, nausea, paleness, sweating, numbness and tingling of the hands or feet, vision blackout or whiteout, and coldness of the skin. The victim might fall to the ground. If a person begins to feel faint, have him or her sit down with the head between the knees or lie down and raise the legs about 12 inches.

Someone who has fainted should be encouraged to stay lying down until he or she awakens and feels better. Raise the feet and legs about 12 inches. Make sure the person's breathing passage (airway) stays open. If the victim begins to vomit while lying down, turn the person onto one side and keep the airway clear. Support the head with a pillow or let the victim rest it on one arm. Loosen clothing around the neck. Wipe the victim's forehead with a cool, wet cloth. If the person is alert enough and might be dehydrated, give fluids to drink. If the person does not awaken within two minutes, or fully recover with a few minutes, get medical help.

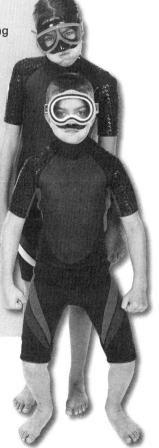

Hyperventilation

Hyperventilation happens when you are breathing faster and deeper than your body needs. *Involuntary (or unintentional) hyperventilation* may be caused by severe pain, infection, severe bleeding, heart attack, cold water immersion, diabetic coma, poisoning, or conditions such as anxiety attacks. The victim can feel dizzy, faint, and numbness, tingling, and cramping in the fingers and toes. Involuntary hyperventilation usually requires immediate medical attention. *Voluntary (or deliberate) hyperventilation* is unhealthy and can be dangerous, especially if it is followed by breath holding. A person who does this can pass out or faint from lack of oxygen before he feels the need to breathe. If this occurs while a person is underwater, the result can be drowning. Be alert to abnormal breathing patterns in individuals.

Loss of Consciousness

Taking too many drugs or drinking too much alcohol can make a person lose consciousness.

Never give an unconscious person anything to drink, throw water on the face, or offer stimulants such as smelling salts. Do not shake or slap the person in an effort to wake him or her up.

A loss of consciousness for more than two minutes is a serious medical condition. An unconscious person might have been hit in the head or had a heart attack or stroke. Diabetics can lose consciousness from either very high or very low blood sugar. Look for an emergency medical ID bracelet or necklace or an information card that identifies health problems such as diabetes. Follow the instructions on the card exactly.

Whenever a person is unconscious for more than a minute or two, call 911 or your local emergency-response number for medical assistance. Check to see if the person is breathing and for other signs of life. Begin CPR if appropriate. If there has been an accident, protect the victim's head and neck from movement.

If the unconscious person has not been involved in an accident, look around the scene for evidence of poisoning, drug use, or other possible causes for the loss of consciousness. If you suspect poison or drugs were involved, take the container or suspected poison to the emergency room with the victim. If the victim recovers before medical personnel arrive, he or she should seek medical advice as soon as possible. *Any loss of consciousness after a head injury, even if only for a short time, requires immediate evaluation by a health-care professional.*

Seizures

A *seizure* is a change in awareness or behavior that is caused by abnormal electrical activity in the brain. In adults and children over age 6, seizures are usually due to epilepsy, a disorder of the brain. A seizure could be a signal of a serious medical problem. Seizures can occur in a person who is suffering from a head injury, brain tumor, stroke, poisoning, electrical shock, heatstroke, infection, a high fever (usually in children), low blood sugar, or low blood pressure.

Epilepsy may be the cause of a seizure. There are several common forms of epilepsy. In *grand mal* epilepsy (also known as tonic/clonic seizure), the victim may lose consciousness and fall to the ground. The arms and legs stiffen then jerk forcefully. Some muscles or the entire body can stiffen or twitch with sudden muscle spasms known as *convulsions.* The victim may bite the tongue. Neck veins may be swollen and the face may turn red or blue. Breathing may decrease and is often loud and labored, accompanied by grunts or snorts with an unusual hissing sound. The victim may drool or foam at the mouth and may lose bladder or bowel control

Another kind of epileptic seizure is the *petit mal* seizure in which the person seems to briefly lose awareness of his or her surroundings and appears to stare into space. This behavior is often mistaken for daydreaming. Although awake, the individual does not respond normally. Afterward, the person does not recall the episode. *Focal* seizures cause one part of the body to jerk or twitch, and the person seems distant or unaware.

While there is no first-aid measure that will stop a seizure, you can provide good first aid by protecting the person from being injured while experiencing a seizure. Break the person's fall, if possible, and lower him or her gently to the floor or ground.

Step 1—Move away any furniture and hard or sharp objects that could cause injury. Avoid moving the person unless there is potential danger nearby—a fireplace, stairway, glass door, swimming pool, or other hazard.

Step 2—Loosen tight clothing around the neck and waist.

Step 3—Do not try to hold the person. Trying to restrain someone during a seizure risks injury to that person and to the first-aider.

Step 4—Do not force anything into the mouth or between the teeth.

Step 5—Make sure the airway remains open.

Step 6—When the seizure is over, place the person in a recovery position.

Step 7—Let the person rest. Keep curious onlookers away.

Step 8—If the person is not known to have epilepsy, if the seizure lasts more than five minutes, recurs, or causes injury, or if the person is slow to recover, call 911 or your local emergency-response number. Call for emergency assistance immediately if a seizure victim is pregnant, diabetic, unconscious, or injured, or has swallowed large amounts of water (as a result of an aquatic accident).

Epilepsy is controlled by medications. While it may not always be necessary to call 911 for a seizure victim who has epilepsy, when in doubt, call 911. Regardless, a seizure victim may still need medical attention.

Recovery Position

Place a victim who is unconscious but who is breathing normally in a recovery position. To do this, extend the person's lower arm, in line with his or her body; support the head and neck as you grasp the victim's hip and shoulder, and roll the person toward you so that he or she is lying on the side. This will prevent the person from choking on saliva, blood (from a bitten tongue), or vomit, and will help keep the airway open. Continue to monitor the person's breathing until medical help arrives.

You may need to turn a person who has been in a recovery position for 30 minutes or longer to the opposite side to stimulate circulation. However, do not move a person with suspected spinal injury unless it is absolutely necessary.

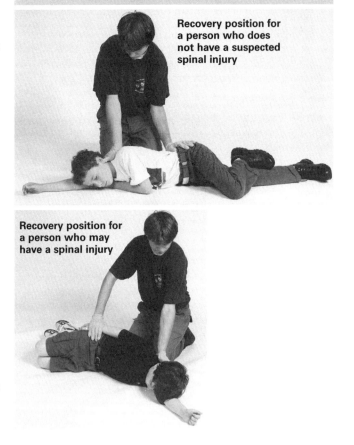

Recovery position for a person who does not have a suspected spinal injury

Recovery position for a person who may have a spinal injury

Diabetes

Diabetes is a disorder that impairs the body's ability to control its blood sugar level. In some cases, the body stops making insulin. Insulin is a hormone that helps the body use sugar for energy. Some people who have diabetes must inject insulin to live. People with diabetes who do not have to use insulin can keep their blood sugar at the proper levels by watching what they eat and taking other diabetes-controlling medications.

When a diabetic person's blood-sugar level is too high or too low, the person can become unconscious. This is a diabetic emergency. A very high blood sugar level *(hyperglycemia)* will rarely cause death; a low blood sugar level *(hypoglycemia)* is extremely dangerous because without sugar, brain cells die quickly and permanent brain damage can result. Because it is impossible to know if there is too much or too little sugar without doing a blood test, all unconscious diabetics should be treated as though their blood sugar levels are too low.

> Warning signals of *hypoglycemia* include headache; sweating; pale, moist skin; weakness; dizziness; shallow breathing; and a rapid pulse. Signals of *hyperglycemia* include extreme thirst, frequent urination, drowsiness, lack of appetite, and labored breathing.

A diabetic person may be wearing a medical ID necklace or bracelet or have a card explaining what should be done during a diabetic emergency. The person might also carry some form of concentrated sugar, to be taken orally if low blood sugar is suspected. Follow the instructions exactly.

Diabetics who use insulin sometimes have a low blood sugar level without becoming unconscious. This can happen if they take too much insulin, don't eat enough food, exercise a lot without eating a snack, or if they decrease their dose of insulin ahead of time or wait too long between meals. With mild cases of hypoglycemia like these (and the victim is fully conscious and able to safely swallow food or drinks), give the victim fruit juice or a soft drink that contains sugar (nondiet).

Hypoglycemia is also called insulin reaction or insulin shock.

Foreign Object in the Eye

Something in the eye is not just painful—it could endanger eyesight. The National Society to Prevent Blindness says that 90 percent of all eye damage is preventable. To protect your eyes, always wear safety glasses or goggles when using power tools, lawn and garden equipment, and other machinery that slings dirt and debris. Be careful not to let fumes from solvents and cleaning agents burn your eyes.

If a foreign object gets in the eye, do not rub the eye; rubbing might scratch the cornea (the clear covering of the colored part of the eye). Have the person blink the eyes; tears might flush out the object. If that doesn't work, wash your hands with soap and water, then try to flush out the foreign particles with clean running water or clean water poured from a glass or bottle.

Foreign matter that is embedded in the eye or that will not wash out must be treated by a physician. Stabilize the object if possible and cover the injured eye with a dry, sterile gauze pad. Take the person to a doctor.

When you are outdoors on windy days, help protect your eyes by wearing sunglasses.

Nosebleeds

Nosebleeds might look bad, but they normally are not very serious and will usually stop in just a few minutes. The bleeding usually stems from a small vein in the nose and can be caused by irritation to the area from colds, allergies, picking, cold and dry weather, and overuse of nose drops or sprays.

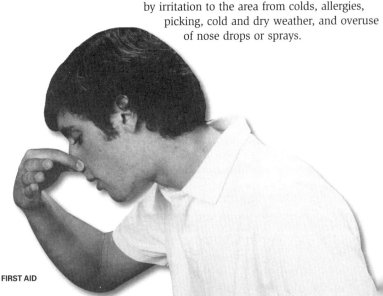

Have the victim sit leaning slightly forward so that the blood does not run down the throat. Ask the person to use thumb and forefinger to pinch the nose firmly but gently, and apply pressure on the upper lip, just below the nose. While the person is pinching, apply a cold compress to the nose and surrounding area.

After about 10 minutes, have the person slowly release the nose pinch. If the bleeding reappears, pinch the nose and apply pressure once again. After the bleeding stops, do not irritate, pick, or blow the nose for several hours. If the bleeding continues for more than 15 minutes, seek medical attention.

For Internal Poisoning, Call 800-222-1222

A poison is a drug, chemical, or toxic liquid that can cause illness or death if swallowed. Any drug or medicine can be poisonous if not taken according to a doctor's instructions or the directions on the label. Many cosmetics, cleaning products, pesticides, paints, and other household products also contain chemicals that may be harmful if swallowed.

Call the Poison Control Center toll-free at 800-222-1222 if you have a poisoning emergency. Keep this number handy. Meanwhile, follow these steps.

Step 1—Immediately take any poison containers to a telephone. Call the poison control center toll-free at 800-222-1222, or 911, or your local emergency response number (if a life-threatening condition such as unconsciousness, a change in consciousness, or no breathing is found), and follow the instructions you are given.

Step 2—Treat the victim for shock and monitor breathing. Do not give anything by mouth unless you are told to do so by medical professionals.

Step 3—Save any vomit (use a bowl, cook pot, or plastic bag). It will help a physician identify the poison and give the right treatment.

Poisonous Plants

Poison Control Center

800-222-1222

The oily sap from the leaves, stem, and roots of poison ivy, poison oak, and poison sumac irritates the skin of most people. Once the sap gets on skin, it can spread to other parts of the body and cause a rash with redness, blisters, swelling, itching, burning, fever, and headache. The severity of the reaction depends on the individual and the extent of the exposure. The best form of prevention is to learn how to recognize the poisonous plants in your area and to avoid contact with them.

Learn what poisonous plants look like and stay away from them. "Leaflets three, let it be" might help you remember to avoid plants that have leaflets grouped in threes, such as poison ivy. White berries are another signal of poisonous plants, although not all plants with three leaves or white berries are poisonous. Wear protective clothing (disposable coveralls, rubber-coated or nonlatex gloves) and take care when handling tools, clothing, and gear that could be contaminated.

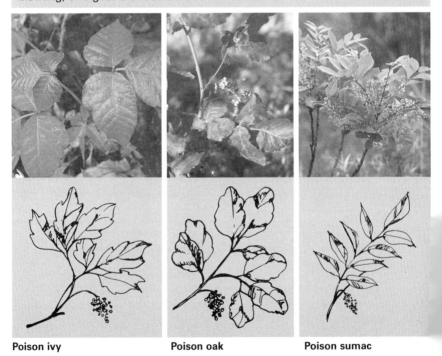

Poison ivy   Poison oak   Poison sumac

The sap of these plants must be on your skin for 10 to 20 minutes before it starts to cause problems. So, if you think you have touched a poisonous plant, immediately stop to wash the exposed area well with soap and water. Wipe with rubbing alcohol and apply calamine or other soothing skin treatment. If the reaction is severe, if the genital area is affected, or if plant parts were chewed or swallowed, seek immediate medical attention.

The sap also binds well to clothing, so change clothes. Keep the outfit you were wearing separate from your other clothing, and wash it separately back home.

Abdominal Pain

There are many causes of abdominal pain. It might be as harmless as an upset stomach or as dangerous as appendicitis. Always take all complaints of abdominal pain seriously. Watch the person closely for increasing pain or changes in the level of consciousness. Most people who have appendicitis will have the same symptoms. First there is a loss of appetite. Then a pain begins in the lower right quarter of the abdomen and gets worse over several hours. Finally, there is nausea and vomiting.

If you think someone might have appendicitis, do not allow the person to eat or drink. Call 911 or a physician immediately. Also seek medical attention if someone suffering abdominal pain has a temperature of 102 degrees or higher or if there are signals of blood in the urine, vomit, or stool.

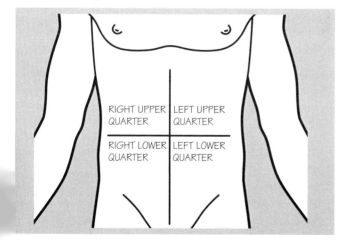

RIGHT UPPER QUARTER | LEFT UPPER QUARTER

RIGHT LOWER QUARTER | LEFT LOWER QUARTER

Dental Injuries

A blow to the face can knock out a tooth or break a jaw. These dental injuries require immediate medical treatment. However, an infected tooth with pain, fever, or swelling can be just as serious and also requires treatment without delay.

Braces and retainers. If a wire is causing irritation, cover the end of the wire with a small cotton ball, beeswax, cold candle wax, or a piece of gauze until you can get the person to the dentist. If a wire is embedded in the cheek, tongue, or gum tissue, do not attempt to remove it. See a dentist or orthodontist immediately.

Bitten lip or tongue. Apply direct pressure to the bleeding area with a clean cloth. If swelling is present, apply a cold, wet cloth or pad. If the bleeding does not stop, the injured person should seek medical attention.

Toothache. Have the victim rinse the mouth vigorously with warm water (to clean out debris); use dental floss to remove any food that might be trapped between the teeth. If swelling is present, place a cold, wet cloth or pad on the outside of the cheek. Have the person see a dentist immediately—toothache may be a signal that infection is present.

Broken, chipped, or loosened tooth. Gently rinse the mouth with warm water. Place a cold, wet cloth or pad in the area of the injury, to minimize swelling. The victim should see a dentist immediately; take the broken or chipped piece of tooth along.

Knocked-out tooth. Pick up the tooth carefully by the crown (not the root). Rinse the tooth gently under cold running water or with milk, if it is available. Do not scrub, scrape, or dry the tooth, and do not allow the tooth to dry. Flush the wound with clean water or saline solution. Apply pressure with a clean cloth or gauze to stop any bleeding. Place the tooth in a container of milk or cool water. Take the victim and the tooth and go directly to the dentist's office or emergency room, ideally within 30 minutes.

Possible fractured jaw. Keep the jaw from moving by using a handkerchief, necktie, towel, or similar item. If swelling is present, apply cold, wet cloths or pads. Call a dentist or take the victim immediately to the emergency room.

Proper dental care and maintenance will prevent many dental injuries. To reduce the chance of tooth injury, follow these tips.

- Always use your safety belt when riding in an automobile.

- Wear the proper safety gear, including a mouth guard, when playing contact sports.

- Never bite down on hard items such as popcorn kernels, ice, or nutshells.

- Do not use your teeth to open packages or bottles.

Do not use heat or place aspirin on an aching tooth or gum tissues.

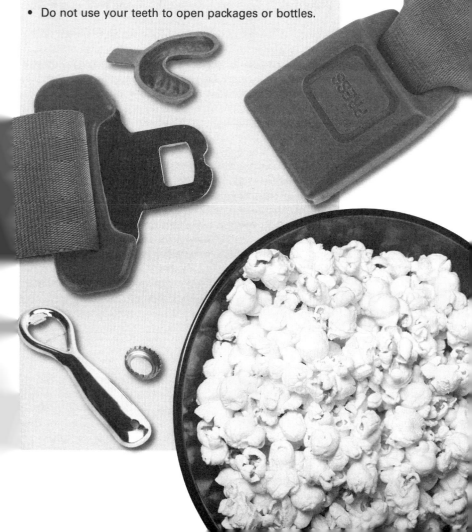

Bites and Stings

The bites of mosquitoes, chiggers, and no-see-ums are irritating but not usually dangerous. More troublesome are ticks, some spiders, and some ants. To avoid getting bitten by **ticks,** wear long pants and a long-sleeved shirt whenever you are in tick-infested woodlands and fields. Button your collar and tuck your pant cuffs into your boots or socks. Inspect yourself daily, especially the hairy parts of your body, and immediately remove any ticks you find.

Ticks bury their heads beneath the skin of their victims. To remove a tick, with gloved hands, grasp it with tweezers close to the skin and gently pull until it comes loose. Don't squeeze, twist, or jerk the tick, as doing so could leave its mouthparts still buried in the skin. Wash the wound with soap and water and apply an antiseptic. Thoroughly wash your hands after handling a tick.

The female **black widow spider** (which is responsible for bites) is glossy black with a red-orange hourglass marking on the underside of its abdomen. These spiders like to dwell under stones and logs, in long grass, brush piles, barns, garages, latrines, and other shadowy spots. Its bite can cause redness and sharp pain, sweating, nausea and vomiting, stomach pain and cramps, and severe muscle pain and spasms. Breathing might become difficult.

When removing a tick, do not burn the tick, prick it with a pin, or cover it with petroleum jelly or nail polish. Doing so may cause the tick to release more of the disease-carrying bacteria.

Black widow spider

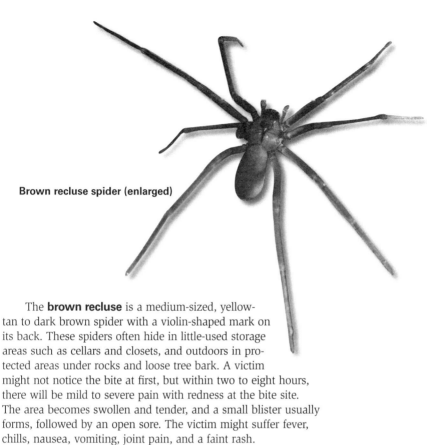

Brown recluse spider (enlarged)

The **brown recluse** is a medium-sized, yellow-tan to dark brown spider with a violin-shaped mark on its back. These spiders often hide in little-used storage areas such as cellars and closets, and outdoors in protected areas under rocks and loose tree bark. A victim might not notice the bite at first, but within two to eight hours, there will be mild to severe pain with redness at the bite site. The area becomes swollen and tender, and a small blister usually forms, followed by an open sore. The victim might suffer fever, chills, nausea, vomiting, joint pain, and a faint rash.

Wash the bite site with soap and water, and apply a cold pack to the area. Seek medical attention immediately.

The sting of a **fire ant** can be extremely painful. If disturbed, fire ants will swarm and attack cooperatively and aggressively, often grabbing hold of the victim's skin and stinging repeatedly. Be careful not to break the tiny blisters that form from the stings. Wash the injured area well, using antiseptic or soap and water. Cover with a sterile bandage and, for relief, try a paste made of baking soda and water, and take a mild nonaspirin pain reliever. The blistered area should heal within a week.

Fire ants live in loose mounds of dirt. If you see such a structure, do not disturb it.

Some people may be highly allergic to fire ant bites, which can cause the life-threatening reaction called *anaphylactic shock (anaphylaxis).* For more information, see "Life-Threatening Emergencies."

If you are stung by a **bee** but are not allergic to bee stings, you can simply remove the stinger by scraping it out with a knife blade. Don't try to squeeze the stinger out. Doing so will force more venom into the skin from the sac attached to the stinger. For bee, wasp, or hornet stings, use an ice pack to help reduce pain and swelling.

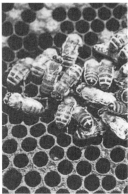 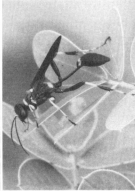 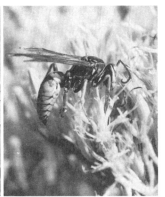

Honeybees   **Mud dauber wasp**   **Paper wasp**

 For information about *anaphylactic shock (anaphylaxis)*, a severe allergic reaction, see "Life-Threatening Emergencies." Without immediate treatment, a person who goes into anaphylactic shock can die. People who are allergic to bee or wasp stings, fire ant bites, or peanuts, shellfish, and certain other foods can have similar anaphylactic reactions. Small children may be especially vulnerable to a severe reaction.

Common scorpion stings often cause severe, sharp pain with swelling and discoloration, but generally cause no lasting ill effects. An ice pack or cold compress should help relieve any itching and pain. An over-the-counter antihistamine may help relieve symptoms. However, if the victim has a history of allergic reactions to insect stings or shows signals of illness, seek medical help at once.

Animal bites. The bite of a dog, cat, or any other warm-blooded animal is a serious puncture wound. The animal might suffer from rabies, a deadly illness that can be transmitted through the saliva of some mammals, in particular dogs, skunks, raccoons, foxes, and bats. The only way to learn if an animal is infected is to catch it and have it tested by medical experts.

An unprovoked attack could be a sign that an animal is rabid. Report all animal bites to your local public health authorities or the police. Do not kill the animal unless necessary, and do not put yourself at risk by trying to catch the animal. Call the police, rangers, or animal control officers, who are trained to do the job safely. Suspicious animals may be confined and observed, or destroyed so that their brains can be tested for rabies.

To treat an animal bite, scrub the area with soap and water and, if possible, flush the wound with clean water for a full five minutes to remove saliva. Control the bleeding and cover the wound with a sterile bandage. The victim **must** see a doctor, who can determine whether to give rabies shots.

If the bite is that of a pet dog or cat, get the name, address, and phone number of the owner, if possible. If bitten by a wild animal, do not try to capture it. Instead, have someone make note of the type of animal, its description, and the direction in which it was headed, then contact the local public health authorities to report the bite.

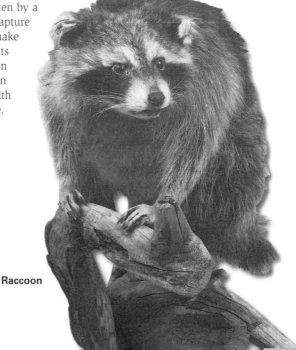

Raccoon

Snakebites. The bite of a nonvenomous snake causes only minor puncture wounds and can be treated as such. Since snakes are not warm-blooded, they cannot carry rabies. Scrub the bite with soap and water, treat with an antiseptic, and cover with a sterile bandage. However, a venomous snakebite requires special care.

The venomous snakes of North America are pit vipers and coral snakes. Pit vipers, including rattlesnakes, copperheads, and cottonmouths, have triangular-shaped heads with pits on each side in front of their eyes. Signals of a pit viper bite include puncture marks, pain (perhaps extreme) and swelling (possibly severe), skin discoloration, nausea and vomiting, shallow breathing, blurred vision, and shock.

Coral snakes have black noses and are marked with red and yellow bands side-by-side, separated by bands of black. They inject a powerful venom that affects the victim's nervous system. The signals of a coral snakebite include slowed physical and mental reactions, sleepiness, nausea, shortness of breath, convulsions, shock, and coma.

The bite of a venomous snake can cause sharp, burning pain. The area around the bite might swell and become discolored; however, a venomous snake does not inject venom every time it bites. Here are the steps for treating the bite of venomous snakes.

Step 1—Get the victim under medical care as soon as possible so that physicians can neutralize the venom.

Step 2—Remove rings and other jewelry that might cause problems if the area around the bite swells.

Step 3—If the victim must wait for medical attention to arrive, wash the wound. If it is a bite of a coral snake, wrap the area snugly (but comfortably) with an elastic roller bandage.

Step 4—Have the victim lie down and position the bitten part lower than the rest of his body. Encourage him to stay calm. He might be very frightened, so keep assuring him that he is being cared for.

Step 5—Treat for shock.

Do not make any cuts on or apply suction to the bite, apply a tourniquet, or use electric shock such as from a car battery. These methods could cause more harm to the victim or are not proven to be effective.

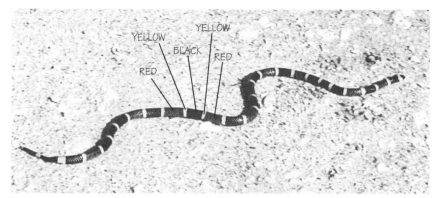

Remember this ditty for safety around coral snakes: red and black—friendly jack; red and yellow–deadly fellow.

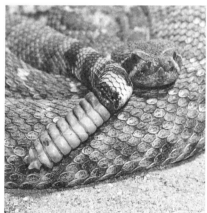

Rattlesnake

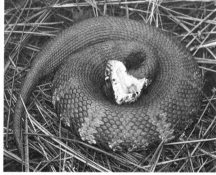

Cottonmouth moccasin

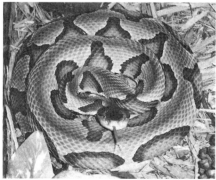

Copperhead

Since nearly all snakebites occur on the limbs, wearing gloves and boots or high leather shoes will protect the most vulnerable areas. The best rule is to never put your feet or hands where you cannot see them. Don't reach over blind hedges or poke around in crevices, hollow logs, or woodpiles.

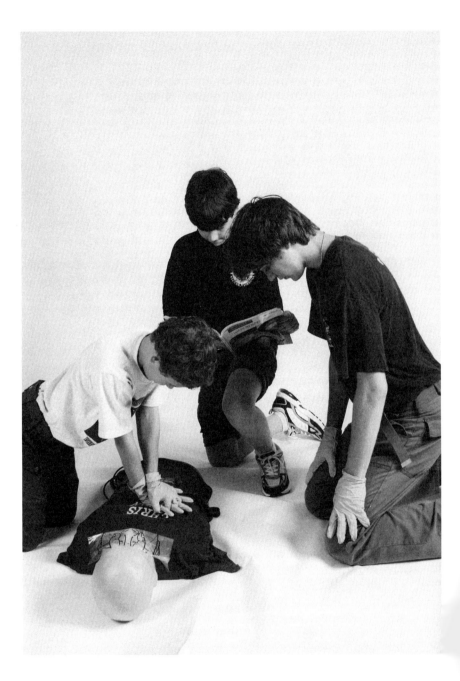

Life-Threatening Emergencies

The right first aid given quickly can save a life. A person who has stopped breathing must receive rescue breathing within three to five minutes or brain damage will occur. People who may need lifesaving first aid include victims of heart attacks, deep cuts with severe bleeding, submersion emergency (or near-drowning), and lightning strikes. After calling for help, assess the situation to decide what you should do and in which order.

Put A-B-C-D Into Practice

Is the person conscious? Tap the person on the shoulder to see if he or she responds. Ask a question such as, "Are you OK?" If there is no response to sound or touch, the person is unconscious. Call or send for medical help.

An easy way to recall the order of treatment in a life-threatening emergency is A-B-C-D: **A**irway, **B**reathing, **C**irculation, and **D**efibrillation.

A Is for Airway

The airway is the passage that allows air entering the mouth or nose to reach the lungs. Always protect the airway of any accident victim. If the person begins to vomit, turn the victim onto his or her side so that the vomit comes out of the mouth and is not aspirated (inhaled) into the lungs.

Learn to recognize life-threatening conditions and be prepared to take quick action. The procedures for adults, children, and infants may differ slightly.

Tilt the head and lift up on the chin to open the airway of an unconscious person.

If opening the airway restores breathing, place the victim in a recovery position. Continue to monitor the person's breathing until help arrives.

If a victim is unconscious, carefully place the person on his or her back, protecting the head and neck if you must roll the person over. Then, open the airway by pressing (or tilting) on the forehead with one hand and lifting the chin with the other to tilt back the head. This action will keep the tongue from blocking the person's airway.

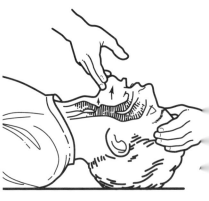

B Is for Breathing

After opening the victim's airway, check to see if the person can breathe normally. Place your cheek in front of the victim's mouth (about 1 to 2 inches away). Look, listen, and feel for movement and breathing (signals of circulation, or "signs of life") for no more than 10 seconds. If the person is breathing effectively, you will feel and hear the airflow on your cheek and see and feel the chest rising and falling at regular intervals. *If there is no breathing or movement; give two rescue breaths, then begin cardiopulmonary resuscitation.*

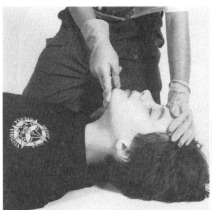
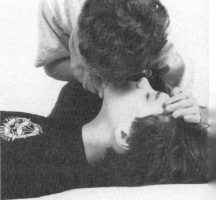

Look, listen, feel—these are the steps to check for breathing.

Once you have opened the airway, check for movement and breathing for no more than 10 seconds. If the person still is not breathing, give two rescue breaths.

Step 1—Place a CPR breathing barrier over the victim's mouth. That may protect both of you from orally transmitted diseases.

Step 2—Give two rescue breaths. While maintaining the head-tilt, pinch the nostrils, seal your mouth over the victim's mouth and blow into it to fill the person's lungs. (For an infant, seal your mouth over both the mouth and nose, then breathe gently.) Each breath should last about 1 second. Watch to see if the chest clearly rises. Remove your mouth and then give another rescue breath.

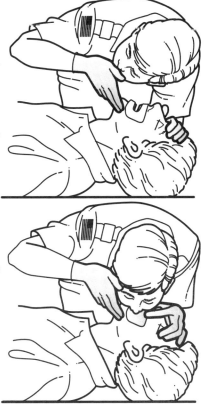

Step 3—For a child or an infant, after two rescue breaths, check for a pulse for no more than 10 seconds. If there is still no breathing, begin rescue breathing (1 breath about every 3 seconds) and recheck for breathing and pulse every 2 minutes as long as there is a pulse but no breathing. **For an adult,** after two rescue breaths, begin CPR immediately if the victim does not resume breathing.

If the victim revives, put him or her in a recovery position and treat for shock. Monitor the person to make sure breathing does not stop again.

Rescue breathing techniques are constantly being improved. Check with your Scout leaders and local American Red Cross chapter or American Heart Association office for current methods and training opportunities.

C Is for Circulation

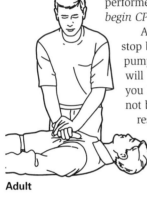

Signals of circulation mean that the heart is still beating and circulating blood through the body. Normal breathing and movement are signals of life and that there is a heartbeat. In the case of young children (under age 12) and infants, feeling for a pulse for no more than 10 seconds can also be performed. *If there are no signals that the heart is beating, begin CPR immediately.*

Accidents or medical conditions that cause a person to stop breathing can also stop the heart. If the heart is not pumping and circulating blood through the body, the victim will not be breathing, moving, or making normal sounds. If you have delivered two rescue breaths and the victim does not begin to breathe, you should perform cardiopulmonary resuscitation, or CPR, immediately.

Learning CPR requires careful instruction from a certified teacher. Perhaps you can practice CPR at Scout meetings. The American Red Cross and American Heart Association offer classes, too. Your Scout leaders can help you find training to learn this lifesaving skill.

Adult

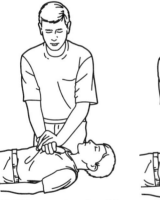
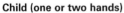

Child (one or two hands)

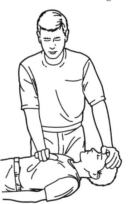
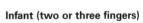

Infant (two or three fingers)

While the techniques for CPR are different for adults, children, and infants, the cycle of 30 chest compressions followed by two rescue breaths applies to everyone. To receive full and proper CPR training, contact your American Red Cross chapter or the American Heart Association. See the resources section in the back of this pamphlet for more information.

D Is for Defibrillation

The heart is made up of many muscle fibers that usually contract and relax in unison to pump blood. During a heart attack, those muscle fibers do not work together. A heart attack can lead to what is known as "cardiac arrest." Another cause of cardiac arrest is an abnormal electrical heart rhythm, most commonly known as ventricular fibrillation.

A machine called a *defibrillator* can send an electrical shock through the heart to momentarily stop all electrical activity. This pause gives the heart enough time to try to restore an effective heartbeat (rhythm). A person whose heart has stopped functioning can be treated with this special device, if one is available. Ideally, this should happen within several minutes of the victim's collapse.

Most ambulances, hospitals, and emergency care facilities are equipped with defibrillators for use by trained medical personnel. Because a defibrillator must be used quickly (within several minutes) to save a person's life, a new type of defibrillator called an *automated external defibrillator (AED)* has been developed. Many first responders such as police officers and firefighters carry and are trained in the use of AEDs.

An AED is computerized. It can check a person's heart rhythm and recognize a rhythm that requires a shock. It can also advise the rescuer when a shock is needed. AEDs use voice prompts, lights, and text messages to tell the rescuer the steps to take.

AEDs are very accurate and easy to use. With only a few hours of training, a layperson can learn how to operate an AED. However, you must be trained to operate one safely and effectively.

Many public places such as airports and shopping malls now have installed AEDs in clearly marked, designated areas much the same way that fire extinguishers are made readily available for access in an emergency.

Heart Attack

Women may experience different symptoms than do men. A woman might also have intermittent back, abdominal, and upper-body pain; unexplained fatigue; and dizziness. She might feel heaviness in the chest or a burning sensation rather than pain.

A heart attack is a life-threatening condition that causes death of or damage to the heart muscle. When an artery that supplies blood to the heart is blocked, a heart attack can occur. Heart attack requires quick action to possibly save a life. Learn to recognize the warning signals of a heart attack, then be prepared to take prompt action by calling 911 or the local emergency-response number. Immediately administer CPR if necessary.

Common Warning Signals of Heart Attack

Here are some common warning signals of heart attack.

- Persistent, uncomfortable pressure, squeezing, fullness, or pain in the center of the chest behind the breastbone. The feeling may spread to the shoulders, arms, and neck. It may last several minutes or longer and may come and go. It need not be severe. (Sharp, stabbing twinges of pain usually are not signals of heart attack.)
- Unusual sweating—for instance, perspiring even though a room is cool.
- Nausea—stomach distress with an urge to vomit.
- Shortness of breath.
- A feeling of weakness.

Should anyone complain of these symptoms, get medical attention for the victim right away. Be aware that a common reaction of men and women who are experiencing signals of heart attack is to deny that anything is wrong. Be ready to begin CPR if the heartbeat and breathing stop.

If you suspect someone is having a heart attack and this person is conscious, try to find out the following.
- Is the person taking any type of blood-thinning medication?
- Is the person allergic to aspirin?
- Does this person have stomach problems?
- Has the person ever been advised by a physician not to take aspirin?

If the answer is "no" to all of the questions above, when you call 911, emergency responders may advise you to offer the person two uncoated baby aspirin tablets (81 mg apiece). Aspirin must be used, not painkillers such as ibuprofen (Advil, Motrin) or acetaminophen (Tylenol).

Stroke

A stroke occurs when an artery to the brain either bursts or is blocked by a clot. When blood supply to the brain is interrupted, brain cells begin to die.

Common Warning Signals of Stroke

This cardiovascular disease injures the brain, and the signals happen fast; the victim might not be aware a stroke is occurring. Others nearby might not know it, either. This is why it is so important to know the common warning signals of stroke.

- Sudden weakness or numbness of the face, arm, or leg (especially on one side of the body)
- Sudden confusion or trouble speaking or understanding speech
- Sudden trouble seeing
- Sudden dizziness, with loss of balance or coordination and trouble walking
- Sudden and severe headache with no known cause

Perhaps someone has suddenly lost the ability to speak clearly or to move one side of the body, or suddenly has trouble walking or seeing. If you think someone is having a stroke, note the last time you saw the person acting normally, then call 911 immediately; fast action is vital.

While waiting for medical personnel to arrive, keep the person calm and comfortable. A stroke could make a person nervous and afraid. Reassure the person that help is on the way. Do not give the victim anything to eat or drink.

Think FAST

Use this quick method to help determine whether someone might have suffered a stroke.

F = Face. Ask the person to smile. Watch for weakness to one side of the face.

A = Arm. Ask the person to raise both arms. Watch for weakness or numbness in the limbs.

S = Speech. Ask the person to say a simple sentence such as, "May I have a cookie?" Listen for slurred speech.

T = Time. Time to call 911 right away if the person cannot perform *any* of the simple tasks above or shows any other signals of stroke. Be sure to note the time the signals began.

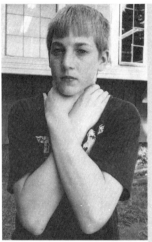

When Someone Is Choking

A person who is choking and can cough, speak, or breathe is still getting some air to the lungs. Encourage him or her to cough up the object, and be ready to administer first aid if it is needed. However, if the person is coughing weakly or making high-pitched noises, or if the person can't cough, speak, or breathe, you will need to take quick action.

Someone who is choking on food may grasp the throat to signal that he or she is unable to breathe. Treat by performing back blows and abdominal thrusts.

Have someone call for help, then do the following.

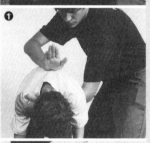

Step 1—If the child or adult is conscious, give a series of five back blows as shown. From behind, place one arm across the person's chest and lean forward. Firmly strike the person's back with the palm of your hand. Follow the five back blows with abdominal thrusts as described in steps 2 and 3.

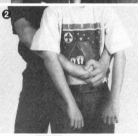

Step 2—Stand behind the victim. Put your arms around the waist and clasp your hands together. The knuckle of one thumb should be just above the victim's navel but below the rib cage.

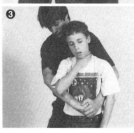

Step 3—Thrust your clasped hands inward and upward with enough force to pop loose the obstruction.

Step 4—Repeat steps 1 through 3 until the obstruction clears or medical help arrives.

Severe Bleeding

A careless moment with a knife, an ax, or a power tool or any number of other accidents can sever a large blood vessel in the arm or leg, causing severe bleeding. Quick first-aid action can stop bleeding and perhaps save a person from bleeding to death.

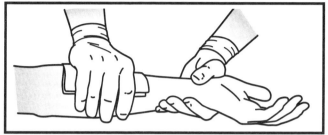

Applying direct pressure on a wound will stop most bleeding.

Wounds can be *incisions*—clean cuts through the skin, such as those caused by knives, razors, broken glass, or other sharp objects, or *lacerations*—rough, jagged cuts. Deep wounds may injure muscles, tendons, and nerves. Contamination of any wound increases the chances of infection.

First Aid for Severe Bleeding

Step 1—Put on nonlatex disposable gloves and protective goggles. With a clean cloth or sterile dressing as a pad, use the palm of your hand to apply firm pressure directly over the wound. If you have an elastic bandage handy, use it to secure the pad tightly over the source of the bleeding.

Step 2—After the bleeding stops, hold the pad in place with a sterile bandage—an athletic wrap, strips torn from clean clothing, or something else similar close at hand. Bind the pad firmly but not so tightly that circulation is cut off.

Step 3—If the bandage is on an arm or a leg, periodically check for circulation (feeling, warmth, color). No circulation is an indication that the bandage should be loosened.

Step 4—If a pressure pad has become soaked with blood, place a fresh pad over the first one (do not remove it) and continue applying pressure.

A paramedic or physician will probably want to know when the injured person was immunized against *tetanus*—a serious illness that can sometimes result when bacteria are introduced through cuts, abrasions, and other breaks in the skin.

TOURNIQUETS

For the most extreme cases of severe bleeding, first-aiders have sometimes used a tourniquet—a device designed specifically to be tightened above a limb that has been partially or completely severed—as a last resort for stopping bleeding. This method is used only when all other efforts have failed and advanced professional medical care is either delayed by at least 30 minutes or not available. A tourniquet will completely stop the flow of blood to the limb. It can also cause gangrene (tissue death) and may require surgical amputation of the limb.

In the past, field tourniquets were made from a strip of cloth at least 2 inches wide (never a cord, wire, rope, or any other thin material). The strip was tied with an overhand knot above the wound, and a stick, tent peg, or similar rod-shaped object was placed on the knot and tied down with a square knot. The stick was then twisted just until the bleeding stopped, and then secured so the tourniquet would not come loose. Today, if a tourniquet must be used, it is generally a commercially made device designed for this specific purpose.

Once a tourniquet has been applied, a written note of the location of the tourniquet and the time it was applied is made and attached to the victim's clothing. The victim should be treated for shock and given first aid for other injuries. The tourniquet must not be covered.

If it is likely that it will be hours before advanced medical help is available, then the tourniquet should be loosened to determine if bleeding has stopped and also to allow some blood flow to the limb after five minutes. If bleeding continues, the tourniquet should be tightened and rechecked after another five-minute period. If the bleeding has stopped, the loosened tourniquet should be left in place. To avoid crushing the tissue and causing permanent damage to nerves and blood vessels, the tourniquet should be periodically checked and loosened.

For any case of severe bleeding, summon emergency medical help immediately. You should always use nonlatex, disposable gloves and protective goggles when rendering aid to a person who is bleeding. Because of the many risks associated with the application of a tourniquet, this method is best left to trained medical professionals or skilled responders specially trained in the application of tourniquets.

If the injury is on a flexible part of the body—an elbow or knee, for example—after the bleeding has stopped, use a splint to immobilize the joint and prevent the wound from pulling open.

Anaphylactic Shock (Anaphylaxis)

For most people, bee or wasp stings will cause pain, redness, and a little swelling around the affected area and perhaps a few days of itching. For the small number of people who are allergic to bee or wasp venom or fire ant bites, these stings and bites can cause a life-threatening reaction called *anaphylactic shock (anaphylaxis)*. Symptoms can include a swelling of throat tissues or tongue that restricts air passages and makes breathing difficult or even impossible.

Without immediate treatment, a person who goes into anaphylactic shock can die. People who are allergic to peanuts, shellfish, and certain other foods can have similar anaphylactic reactions if they ingest or even inhale particles of these foods. For instance, people who are allergic to peanuts cannot consume foods cooked in peanut oil.

Any Scout who has an allergy that could cause anaphylactic shock should share that information with Scout leaders and always let group leaders know where he carries anaphylaxis medications so that they can be made available at a moment's notice.

First Aid for Anaphylactic Shock

Step 1—Call 911 or your local emergency-response number.

Step 2—Check the victim for a medical ID bracelet, necklace, or information card. Ask if the person is carrying a prescribed emergency medical kit. You may be able to assist the person under certain circumstances AND if you are trained and allowed to assist by state or local regulations. If so, follow the kit instructions exactly and assist the person by locating the medication kit and handing it to him or her. It is best that the individual administers the medication. If the person is unconscious, follow the A-B-C-D lifesaving sequence and/or follow instructions provided by emergency medical professionals.

Step 3—See that the victim receives follow-up medical treatment.

If you are not qualified to administer epinephrine, you should help make sure the person stays in a comfortable position for breathing while awaiting medical help. This will usually be a sitting position.

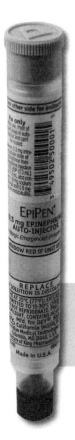

Life-threatening food allergies are rare. However, an increasing number of people suffer from food-allergy reactions that, although not life-threatening, can cause great discomfort. If you have a food allergy, always be sure to let Scout leaders know about it. They can then work with members of the patrol and troop to ensure that the foods that trigger an allergic reaction are avoided during the planning and carrying out of Scout events. Making a situation safe for everyone is also a way to increase the sense of cooperation and support within a Scout unit.

People who know they are susceptible to anaphylaxis should carry emergency kits that contain an injection of epinephrine, a rapidly acting hormone that reverses the effects of anaphylactic shock.

First-Aid Resources

Scouting Literature

Boy Scout Handbook and *Fieldbook; Dentistry, Emergency Preparedness, Fire Safety, Lifesaving, Medicine, Public Health, Safety,* and *Wilderness Survival* merit badge pamphlets

Visit the Boy Scouts of America's official retail Web site (with your parent's permission) at *http://www.scoutstuff.org* for a complete listing of all merit badge pamphlets and other helpful Scouting materials and supplies.

Books

American College of Emergency Physicians First Aid Manual, 2nd ed. DK Publishing, 2003.

American Medical Association Handbook of First Aid and Emergency Care, revised ed. Random House, 2000.

Auerbach, Paul S. *Medicine for the Outdoors: The Essential Guide to Emergency Medical Procedures and First Aid.* Lyons Press, 2003.

Backer, Howard, et al. *Wilderness First Aid: Emergency Care for Remote Locations.* Jones and Bartlett, 2005.

First Aid, 4th ed. American Academy of Orthopaedic Surgeons, 2005.

Forgey, William. *Wilderness Medicine: Beyond First Aid,* 5th ed. Globe Pequot Press, 1999.

Gill, Paul G. *Wilderness First Aid: A Pocket Guide.* Ragged Mountain Press, 2002.

Isaac, Jeffrey. *The Outward Bound Wilderness First-Aid Handbook,* revised ed. Lyons & Burford, 1998.

Rickey, Brad, and Kurt Duffens. *FastAct Pocket First Aid Guide.* FastAct, 1999.

Schimelpfenig, Todd, and Linda Lindsey. *NOLS Wilderness First Aid,* 3rd ed. National Outdoor Leadership School and Stackpole Books, 2000.

Tilton, Buck. *Backcountry First Aid and Extended Care,* 4th ed. Falcon, 2002.

Weiss, Eric A. *Wilderness 911: A Step-by-Step Guide for Medical Emergencies and Improvised Care in the Backcountry.* The Mountaineers Books, 1998.

Wilkerson, James A., ed. *Medicine for Mountaineering and Other Wilderness Activities,* 5th ed. The Mountaineers Books, 2001.

Organizations and Web Sites

American Heart Association
7272 Greenville Ave.
Dallas, TX 75231
Toll-free telephone: 800-242-8721
Web site: *http://www.americanheart.org*

American Medical Association
515 N. State St.
Chicago, IL 60610
Toll-free telephone: 800-621-8335
Web site: *http://www.ama-assn.org*

American Red Cross
2025 E St. NW
Washington, DC 20006
Telephone: 202-303-4498
Web site: *http://www.redcross.org*

American Stroke Association
7272 Greenville Ave.
Dallas, TX 75231
Toll-free telephone: 888-478-7653
Web site:
http://www.strokeassociation.org

National Safety Council
1121 Spring Lake Drive
Itasca, IL 60143-3201
Toll-free telephone: 800-621-7619
Web site: *http://www.nsc.org*

The American Red Cross produces several resources that may be of particular interest to Scouts, Scout leaders, and merit badge counselors.

American Red Cross. *First Aid/CPR/ AED for Schools and the Community* (participant's manual). Staywell, 2006.

American Red Cross. *First Aid/CPR/ AED for Schools and the Community* (DVD). Staywell, 2006.

American Red Cross. *American Red Cross First Aid—Responding to Emergencies* (participant's manual). Staywell, 2007.

American Red Cross. *American Red Cross Sport Safety Training Handbook.* Staywell, 2007.

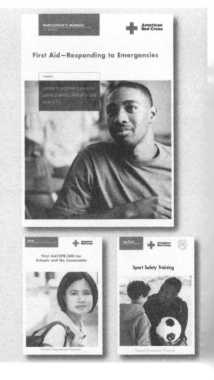

Acknowledgments

For this revision of the *First Aid* merit badge pamphlet, the Boy Scouts of America is grateful to Richard Thomas, Pharm.D., Scottsdale, Arizona, for his thorough reviews and input. Dr. Thomas is a longtime, avid supporter of Scouting who has provided his subject expertise for a number of merit badge pamphlets. We are grateful to Murphy Green, M.D., Harlan, Kentucky, for his early involvement.

Thanks also to the BSA Health and Safety Committee, in particular committee chair George Allen, M.D.; and members Calvin Banning; David Cohen, M.D.; Stephen Lomber, M.D., Ph.D.; and Harold Yocum, M.D.

We appreciate the Quicklist Consulting Committee of the Association for Library Service to Children, a division of the American Library Association, for its assistance with updating the resources section of this merit badge pamphlet.

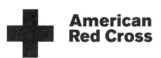 **American Red Cross**

The Boy Scouts of America is grateful to the American Red Cross for providing hands-on assistance from beginning to end with this edition of the *First Aid* merit badge pamphlet. From the text to photos and illustrations, subject expertise, and a multitude of other lines of support, the American Red Cross has been indispensable, professional, and obliging in every way. In particular, the BSA would like to thank the following individuals from the American Red Cross National Headquarters, Preparedness and Health and Safety Services: Ted T. Crites, CHES, manager, Technical Development, First Aid, CPR/AED Programs, Research and Product Development; John E. Hendrickson, senior associate, Program Management and Field Support; and Kate Tunney, M.A.Ed., CHES, senior associate, Technical Development, Research and Product Development.

Photo and Illustration Credits